D1569369

DEMENTIA

Dementia: The Basics provides the reader with a clear and compassionate introduction to dementia and an accessible guide to dealing with different parts of the dementia journey, from pre-diagnosis and diagnosis to post-diagnostic support, increasing care needs and end of life care.

Co-authored by an academic, a person living with dementia and a family carer, the book endeavours to raise awareness of dementia, challenge stereotypical and negative ideas about what it means to have dementia and champion a society where people living with dementia can be as active as they wish for as long as possible. The authors present an overview of current research at each step of the dementia journey as well as including knowledge from lived experience, enhancing understanding and challenging thinking about what it might be like to live with a diagnosis or to care for a loved one. As a whole, the book emphasises the importance of prioritising the person living with dementia, as well as considering the impact of what any initiative or action might mean for them, their families and their care supporters.

Offering both an accessible introduction to dementia and practical tools, this book will be ideal for health and social care professionals, students of social care, health care and nursing, people with dementia, carers and anyone wanting to understand more about the condition.

Anthea Innes, BA, MSc, PhD, is Professor of Dementia and Coles-Medlock Director of the Salford Institute for Dementia, University of Salford, UK. She is a social scientist who has specialised in researching the experiences of dementia and how to bring about change and improvements in dementia care for the last 25 years.

Lesley Calvert lives with Alzheimer's disease and is an associate at the Salford Institute for Dementia, UK. She is a member of the local Dementia Champions Group and a facilitator at the Open Doors Network in Salford. She is also part of the 3 Nations Dementia Working Group.

Gail Bowker has been an unpaid carer since 2010. She is a strong voice in the dementia arena in Greater Manchester, UK, and sits on several local strategic boards and committees. She is a passionate advocate for carers' rights.

The Basics

The Basics is a highly successful series of accessible guidebooks which provide an overview of the fundamental principles of a subject area in a jargon-free and undaunting format.

Intended for students approaching a subject for the first time, the books both introduce the essentials of a subject and provide an ideal springboard for further study. With over 50 titles spanning subjects from artificial intelligence (AI) to women's studies, *The Basics* are an ideal starting point for students seeking to understand a subject area.

Each text comes with recommendations for further study and gradually introduces the complexities and nuances within a subject.

EDUCATION RESEARCH
MICHAEL HAMMOND WITH JERRY WELLINGTON

FINANCE (THIRD EDITION)
ERIK BANKS

FINANCIAL ACCOUNTING
ILIAS G. BASIOUDIS

FOLKLORE
SIMON J. BRONNER

FORENSIC PSYCHOLOGY
SANDIE TAYLOR

GERONTOLOGY
JENNY R. SASSER AND HARRY R. MOODY

GENDER (SECOND EDITION)
HILARY LIPS

JAPAN
CHRISTOPHER P. HOOD

LANGUAGE (SECOND EDITION)
R.L. TRASK

MEN AND MASCULINITY
NIGEL EDLEY

MEDIA STUDIES (SECOND EDITION)
JULIAN MCDOUGALL AND CLAIRE POLLARD

MEDIEVAL LITERATURE
ANGELA JANE WEISL AND ANTHONY JOSEPH CUNDER

MODERNISM
LAURA WINKIEL

NUMERICAL COGNITION
ANDRÉ KNOPS

NARRATIVE
BRONWEN THOMAS

POETRY (THIRD EDITION)
JEFFREY WAINWRIGHT

POVERTY
BENT GREVE

THE QUR'AN (SECOND EDITION)
MASSIMO CAMPANINI

RESEARCH METHODS (SECOND EDITION)
NICHOLAS WALLIMAN

SEMIOTICS
DANIEL CHANDLER

SPECIAL EDUCATIONAL NEEDS AND DISABILITY (THIRD EDITION)
JANICE WEARMOUTH

SPORT MANAGEMENT
ROBERT WILSON AND MARK PIEKARZ

SPORTS COACHING
LAURA PURDY

TRANSLATION
JULIANE HOUSE

TOWN PLANNING
TONY HALL

WOMEN'S STUDIES (SECOND EDITION)
BONNIE G. SMITH

For a full list of titles in this series, please visit www.routledge.com/The-Basics/book-series/B

DEMENTIA

THE BASICS

Anthea Innes, Lesley Calvert
and Gail Bowker

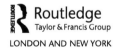

Routledge
Taylor & Francis Group

LONDON AND NEW YORK

First published 2021
by Routledge
2 Park Square, Milton Park, Abingdon, Oxon OX14 4RN

and by Routledge
52 Vanderbilt Avenue, New York, NY 10017

Routledge is an imprint of the Taylor & Francis Group, an informa business

British Library Cataloguing-in-Publication Data
A catalogue record for this book is available from the British Library

Library of Congress Cataloging-in-Publication Data
Names: Innes, Anthea, author.
Title: Dementia : the basics / Anthea Innes, Lesley Calvert, and Gail Bowker.
Description: Milton Park, Abingdon, Oxon ; New York, NY : Routledge, 2020. |
    Series: The basics series | Includes bibliographical references and index.
Identifiers: LCCN 2020011146 (print) | LCCN 2020011147 (ebook) |
    ISBN 9781138897755 (hardback) | ISBN 9781138897762 (paperback) |
    ISBN 9781315709000 (ebook)
Subjects: LCSH: Dementia.
Classification: LCC RC521 .I547 2020 (print) | LCC RC521 (ebook) |
    DDC 616.8/31—dc23
LC record available at https://lccn.loc.gov/2020011146
LC ebook record available at https://lccn.loc.gov/2020011147

ISBN: 978-1-138-89775-5 (hbk)
ISBN: 978-1-138-89776-2 (pbk)
ISBN: 978-1-315-70900-0 (ebk)

Typeset in Bembo
by Apex CoVantage, LLC

Anthea Innes dedicates this work to her grandmother, May Locke.

Lesley Calvert dedicates this work to Sam, her late husband, who *even when he was dying made sure that there was help from family friends and services to keep me as well as possible*.

Gail Bowker dedicates this work to her mother, Geraldine Bowker. Sadly, just after submitting this book to the publisher, Ron, Gail's Dad, passed away. She also dedicates this work to his memory.

CONTENTS

ACKNOWLEDGEMENTS

Our thanks go to Chris Sewards, Megan Wyatt and Sarah Smith for their feedback on individual chapters, and Lesley Waring for her administrative assistance. Innes would also like to acknowledge the discussions with Dr. Fiona Kelly in the development of the original proposal for this book that have informed this iteration.

INTRODUCTION

This book is entitled *Dementia: The Basics* and it aims to do what it says on the tin and provide the reader with an overview of the basics in relation to dementia.

What is dementia, you might be wondering? The World Health Organisation defines dementia as:

> an umbrella term for several diseases that are mostly progressive, affecting memory, other cognitive abilities and behaviour, and that interfere significantly with a person's ability to maintain the activities of daily living.
>
> (2017, 5)

Although the symptoms of dementia may be similar, how one experiences these symptoms and the impact on daily life can vary hugely. The word *disease* might not always be the best word to describe dementia, as dementia is a set of symptoms that develop due to an underlying neurological impairment, in other words, when something begins to happen in the brain. The form of neurological impairment, that is, the part of the brain affected, will relate to the former ability and functioning that may become difficult. Whilst some forms of dementia progress rapidly, many progress at a much slower rate. Anti-dementia medicines can help to slow the progression of dementia, although they do not provide a cure. Other medicines can lead to more acute episodes of dementia symptoms, as can other infections and health issues.

In 2005 an international consensus report estimated that there were 24.3 million people worldwide living with dementia, with an additional 4.6 million new diagnoses per year (Ferri et al., 2005). More recent data from 2015 estimated that there were 46.8 million people with dementia internationally, with 9.9 million new cases per year (Alzheimer Disease International, 2015). Thus the number of people impacted by dementia across the globe is rising and will continue to rise into the twenty-first century due to people living longer and the use of more sophisticated diagnostic processes (Alzheimer Disease International, 2015). Policy drivers to improve diagnosis have accelerated the rising numbers of people identified with dementia. Thirty-three countries now have a national dementia strategy (Alzheimer Disease International, 2018). This demonstrates that more people will experience dementia, and that this is something that is happening across the world. Therefore, regardless of where you might live, the number of people who have dementia is set to rise.

The book has seven chapters. Each chapter deals with different areas of the dementia journey as presented in Figure 0.1.

Chapter 1 focuses on pre-diagnosis. This is the time when an individual may be concerned that something is not quite 'right' or when family members and friends are concerned but do not know what is going on. Chapter 2 talks about the diagnosis of dementia with specific attention of the experience of receiving a diagnosis. We then move on to discuss in chapter 3 issues surrounding post-diagnostic support, that is, things that can be done to support the person with dementia and their family to adapt and to live well with dementia. The chapter discusses increased care and support

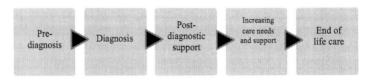

Figure 0.1 The Dementia Journey

needs for the person living with dementia. This may involve receiving a more intensive package of support to enable the person with dementia to remain living in their own home, or it may involve moving into assisted living or care home settings. This can be a challenging period for everyone involved on an emotional level as both the person with dementia and their care supporters adjust to the changing needs and how these might best be met. Chapter 4 considers the support needs of family members and other supporters. Chapter 5 discusses how support can be provided to both the person living with dementia and their care supporters together. Chapter 6 considers the transitions during the journey with dementia as post-diagnostic needs change and develop over time. Chapter 7 focuses on end of life care.

The book is written by three people with very different backgrounds, but with a common purpose: to raise awareness of dementia, to challenge stereotypical and negative ideas about what it means to have dementia and to champion a society where people living with dementia can be as involved as actively as they wish for as long as possible. Innes is a Professor of dementia and has been doing research, education and awareness-raising work about dementia since 1995. Her maternal grandmother, May, had a Parkinson's disease–related dementia and she has been influenced by the experiences and devotion of her family who ensured that May continued to live at home, as was her wish, until her death, at home, in 1993. Calvert is a woman living with dementia, a former district nurse who had provided care to people living with many conditions, including dementia, and who is currently an active member of many dementia groups and organisations. She is a self-proclaimed agitator – she wants to improve dementia services and society to enable people who have dementia to live as well as they can with their dementia for as long as possible. Bowker, a former senior civil servant, has been the primary carer for the last four years for her father, Ron, who has vascular dementia, visual impairment and mobility issues. Prior to this she supported Ron in caring for her mother, who was diagnosed with dementia in 2010 and who passed away in 2017. Bowker is an activist who wants to ensure that people living with dementia and their family members get the best possible care and support available, wherever they live. She represents carers in many regional groups and actively campaigns to ensure that people living with dementia are not forgotten when it comes to designing services and support in her area. From professional and personal experiences, then, all three authors have a passion and commitment to maximising the opportunities available to people diagnosed with dementia to live as well as possible and to challenge stereotypes and bring about change and improvements when required on the basis of research evidence and lived experiences. We provide an overview of the evidence and knowledge that we have based on research and lived experiences. This is important, and our message is clear: please remember to consider what any initiative or action might mean for the person living with dementia and their families and care supporters.

We hope this book will enhance your understanding of dementia, and perhaps challenge your thinking about dementia, in particular, what it might be like to live with a diagnosis of dementia, or provide care to a loved one with dementia. We also hope that it will provide you with some ideas and tips that you might be able to adapt and implement in your particular situation; be it as a health and social care professional, a student who is learning about dementia in relation to whatever course you might be studying, a person with dementia, a carer or someone who has an interest in the subject. Dementia will affect one in three of us, either as someone who will be diagnosed or someone who will provide support to someone with dementia. We can all do something if we encounter a person with dementia. For example, one very simple thing that we can all do is to learn to take time and to ensure we include the person in conversation, rather than perhaps talk over them and ask whoever might be with them. We can also think about our own preconceptions about what dementia is and what it might mean, and think about how we would like to live and be treated by others if we ever experience this condition. We can also remember that even though the person has dementia, they are still first and foremost a person, with a wealth of life experiences, interests and unique personalities. We believe that dementia is something that deserves policy, practice, research and society's attention. We hope you will rise to our challenge and consider what you can do to contribute to a more dementia-supportive society, however basic your contribution may be.

Some facts about dementia

- There are currently around 850,000 people with dementia in the UK.
- There are over 16,000 younger people with dementia in the UK.
- There are over 11,500 people with dementia from black and minority ethnic groups in the UK.
- There will be over a million people with dementia by 2025.
- Two-thirds of people with dementia are women.
- The proportion of people with dementia doubles for every five-year age group.
- One-third of people over 95 have dementia.
- Around 60,000 deaths a year are directly attributable to dementia.
- Delaying the onset of dementia by five years would reduce deaths directly attributable to dementia by around 30,000 a year.
- The financial cost of dementia to the UK is over £26 billion a year.
- Family carers of people with dementia save the UK over £11 billion a year.
- Around 70 percent of people living in care homes have a form of dementia.
- Two-thirds of people with dementia live in the community while one-third live in a care home.

Alzheimer's Society www.alzheimers.org.uk [accessed 11 November 2019]

REFERENCES

Alzheimer Disease International (2015) *World Alzheimer Report 2015 the Global Impact of Dementia an Analysis of Prevalence, Incidence, Cost and Trends.* London: Alzheimer Disease International. www.alz.co.uk/research/WorldAlzheimerReport2015.pdf

Alzheimer Disease International (2018) *From Plan to Impact Progress towards Targets of the Global Action Plan on Dementia.* London: Alzheimer Disease International. www.alz.co.uk/adi/pdf/from-plan-to-impact-2018.pdf?2

Ferri, C.P. Prince, M., Brayne, C. et al. (2005) Global prevalence of Dementia: A Delphi consensus study. *The Lancet* 366(9503):2112–2117.

World Health Organisation (2017) *Global Action Plan on the Public Health Response to Dementia 2017–2025.* https://apps.who.int/iris/bitstream/handle/10665/259615/9789241513487-eng.pdf;jsessionid=C59B0EE5AC4578CB32AD5D2897E54C46?sequence=1

SECTION 1
THE DIAGNOSTIC PROCESS

This section of the book has two chapters. Chapter 1 discusses the early signs and symptoms before a diagnosis is made (what is called *pre-diagnosis*), before moving on in chapter 2 to discuss diagnosis itself.

1

PRE-DIAGNOSIS

Realising that something is wrong or 'not right' is a common experience for people who are concerned about no longer being able to remember things, or having difficulties doing activities they used to be able to do with ease. People may assume this is due to stress, changes in circumstances or 'just part of getting older'. Sometimes it may well be, but it may also be the early signs and symptoms of dementia (Alzheimer Society n.d.). The only way to know for sure is to seek help and advice, most commonly in the first instance from your local doctor, general practitioner or physician.

There has been an increased policy drive internationally (Alzheimer Disease International, 2017) for people living with dementia to help support the move for individuals to receive an earlier diagnosis and local strategies and implementation plans to help make these drivers a reality (Department of Health, 2012, 2016). Achieving earlier detection poses challenges, as until a person approaches health and social care professionals about their concerns they are 'hidden' from the system that opens the door to a diagnosis and post-diagnostic support.

There may be a process of recognition that there is an issue that needs to be addressed. Steeman et al. (2006) outline the processes involved for a person when cognitive changes occur:

Initial awareness

In the very early days of dementia the person affected gradually becomes aware that there is some kind of change, this may present as an intuitive feeling. At this point the common responses can be to normalise (it's just old age), minimise (it's just one thing I can't remember) or excuse any lapses in memory that may occur (I can't remember that detail, that holiday, that person because it was a long time ago, I am tired).

Suspicion

As time passes the person begins to think that something may be wrong particularly where the difficulties become more frequent, noticeable or start affecting everyday life. For some this may be a slow and personal realisation, for others it may be more sudden especially when confronted by the concerns of other people. At this point frustration, uncertainty, fear and stress may be experienced and individuals become hyper-vigilant of how they are able to function.

Suffering in silence

Many people may try to hide changes from others, to work apart from even those closest to them and effectively to 'suffer in silence'. It is a time when individuals come to a realisation that something significant is happening but the fear and psychological stress may prevent opening up to others. Sometimes experiences cannot be hidden from close family and friends and it may be that their concern or frustration leads to a quest for information.

These changes in cognitive abilities are likely to be observed by family members and friends of the person and all contribute to a time where all those involved feel concern, puzzlement, frustration, anxiety or denial (Robinson, 2010; Jackson, 2010). It has been long recognised that cognitive changes can be subtle and difficult to identify (Clark et al., 2003). Families and the person directly affected may choose not to tell others due to fear, embarrassment or the awareness of the stigma that can accompany memory difficulties (Kim et al., 2019; Alzheimer Disease International, 2012). Some may believe that beyond their immediate families and their communities may not be supportive of their difficulties and they fear other people's reactions (McCleary et al., 2013).

A recent review by Perry-Young et al. (2018) found that the changes people experience are responded to in one of three ways: (1) they discount them as normal, (2) they reserve judgement as to there cause and significance or (3) they misattribute them. In this way there are ongoing delays in seeking help. In a Canadian study, the person with the memory problem was often more aware and aware earlier than their family members that something was not quite right. However, the initial symptoms of dementia were perceived as ambiguous and were often normalised and attributed to other health problems, leading to periods of one to two years where no action to seek help was taken (Leung et al., 2011). It can be seen, then, that individuals with concerns and their family members often seek to 'explain away' what is happening as general ageing or personality issues, which can delay their seeking help. In the case of some minority groups, this misattribution of the underlying cause of issues experienced has been reported as leading to a delay of up to four years before seeking help (McCleary et al., 2013).

Even when someone does take the step and raises with health professionals that they believe something is 'wrong' or 'not right', there is not always a quick or easy answer. A period of investigation often begins, to rule out what may be causing the problems, as well as to work out what is causing the problems. This can mean trips to clinics, hospitals, tests, questions and contact with different professionals. All the while this means waiting, and often worrying, by the person who ultimately receives the diagnosis and their family.

Early diagnosis has long been argued to be the first step in providing an early intervention to older people and their families when they first suspect that something may be 'wrong' (National Audit Office, 2007). Early detection, diagnosis and intervention for people with dementia and their carers may also help reduce costs and improve quality of future care (Prince et al., 2016). Early detection and diagnosis provides a range of opportunities for primary care teams to respond to the potential needs of people with dementia and their caregivers, including prescribing anti-dementia drugs; collecting and processing information about the condition; and beginning to think about possible support needs and service input that may be required to support the person with dementia and their family to continue to live in the community. It is these factors that have led to the development of dementia strategies across the globe (Alzheimer

Disease International, 2017) (at the time of writing, 33 countries have dementia strategies or plans), all of which have early detection at their core. Primary care teams, that is, doctors, nurses and other allied health professionals, are often the first contact point for many people with dementia and their families. It is crucial that members of such teams have a high awareness of the symptoms of dementia and can assist in detecting possible cases of dementia. This is not always easy. A challenge for early diagnosis, and consequentially, early interventions, has been that many general practitioners doubt the benefits of early diagnosis (Woods et al., 2003), not because they do not see the value of a diagnosis, but due to concerns about, for example, the lack of available support and services following a diagnosis (Giezendanner, 2019).

Family members and friends may recognise changes in the abilities, mood and overall wellbeing of the person. Family and friends may try compensate for this by taking on tasks in the family that were traditionally carried out by the person now having problems, for example, paying bills or sending out birthday cards to other family members. Or they may try to assist the person, for example, by going shopping to ensure that essentials are purchased or to the bank to ensure that cash is paid in or withdrawn correctly. The person concerned about their abilities may also adopt strategies to cope and adapt with the issues they are experiencing, or they may put their experiences down to stress, getting older or another health condition that may be causing them difficulties.

Because of the tendency to look for other explanations, or to find ways to compensate for difficulties, there is often a delay in asking for help and seeking the input from health professionals such as the GP or district nurse. By the time the person or their family is really concerned and approaches health services for help they are often frustrated by a delay in the process of being screened, assessed and eventually receiving a diagnosis.

There have been increasing calls for earlier treatment for people living with dementia that have led, for example, to a UK policy drive to explore how best to screen for factors that may be present pre-diagnosis of dementia – although it has been argued that this is not necessarily evidence based and that it is a policy response rather than a clinically driven response (Le Couteur et al., 2013). In Canada (Chertkow et al., 2013) there has also been a focus on the pre-dementia states to find a way to provide an earlier diagnosis. However, Lilford and Hughes (2018) demonstrate that scientific work exploring the biomarkers that could help identify who might be at risk of different forms of dementia pose ethical issues in practice, as not everyone with the biomarkers may go on to have dementia and the support available to those who may be effected would be limited. They therefore do not recommend this approach beyond a research setting. The scientific community is therefore active in seeking to identify factors that may lead to an earlier diagnosis. Yet, there is evidence that screening for memory loss identifies less than one in five of those who will subsequently develop dementia (Palmer et al., 2003). Pre-diagnosis screening has further been argued (Illiffe, 2015) to have negligible benefit to those living with dementia. The research relating to pre-diagnosis therefore is largely exploratory to identify potential risk factors and biomarkers indicating potential dementia.

The research evidence on the experience of pre-diagnosis for those with concerns about their wellbeing is relatively limited. The policy drive to provide earlier screening and support is however understandable given the difficulties that have been reported in receiving a diagnosis. For example, how long it takes, how it is given and the lack of follow-up support offered and/or services available (as we will discuss in detail in chapter 3, post-diagnostic support). Recent work in England demonstrates that those who eventually are given a diagnosis of dementia reduce their social engagement, both in person and via the telephone, compared to people who do not develop dementia in the two years leading up to their diagnosis (Hackett et al., 2019). The experiences of people, and the changes in their patterns and level of social interactions and engagement may be in direct response to how they are coping with early signs and symptoms of dementia, and also how others respond to them. Perry-Young et al.'s (2018) review demonstrates that it is not until there is an event that prompts a need for help that advice and input is sought and received. It is the *impact* on people's lives and those around them, which can be seen as social factors rather than clinical factors, that is of most concern to us here in this book. This is also the primary issue for those who are concerned about their health and who are beginning to seek an explanation as to why they can no longer remember someone's name or how to complete a task, for example.

It was the response of co-workers to one of the authors of this book that led her to seeking help in identifying what might be happening to her.

Lesley's story, as a younger person who was working when she started to experience problems with memory and functioning at work, exemplifies the difficulties in recognising and acknowledging that there is a problem and to identify what the problem might be.

Lesley's Story

I started my nurse training in 1970 at the age of 18 and worked for Salford since I qualified, first as a nurse at Hope Hospital until 1975 and then as a district nurse. I was a competent nurse and like the rest of the team I was able to multitask, something all nurses are expected to do. I could remember the names and addresses and what I needed to do for the patients I was to visit each evening, without looking in my diary. I could remember everything I had done for each patient without writing it down. However, in January 2013 I began to notice that I was having difficulty. These are the problems I was having:

1   Remembering the names of common things or where I had put them.
2   Forgetting how to do nursing procedures that I had done competently for many years.
3   Getting lost driving to patients' homes that I had visited for a number of years.
4   Unable to document the care I had given to a patient and to write a comprehensive sentence. I wrote in one patients' nursing notes and not one sentence made sense. As these notes are legal documents this really worried me.
5   Unable to finish a conversation.
6   Losing my train of thought or being unable to remember what I was saying if I was interrupted.

One night it was like the game 'give us a clue' when you had to guess what I had done, but I couldn't remember; each nurse tried to help me by saying a word. Eventually one nurse mentioned the word I was looking for and it registered in my brain and I got a round of applause.

Alarm bells were ringing but I was getting older and the workload was increasing. I thought it was a combination of stress and old age.

Probably, looking back, the problem had been going on for over a year as I'd had numerous disagreements with my mother and others when they had said they had told me something and I had insisted they hadn't, or they would say to me, you've told me that three times and I would say I hadn't. I obviously had not remembered.

One evening in January I did something out of character: I threw a book at one of my colleagues when she told me I had told her the same thing three times. I didn't remember telling her once, let alone three times.

I decided it was time to visit the doctor. I told her my concerns and she, like me, thought it was stress related but decided to check my blood and I also had an ECG (electro-cardiogram). On my return I was expecting her to tell me I had a thyroid problem or something else that could cause the memory problems, but she told me all my results were normal. My heart sank, I shed a few tears, as we had nursed my dad with Alzheimer's until his death at the age of 68. He was diagnosed in his late fifties. I had also nursed my grandmother with Alzheimer's and the signs I was showing were the same but not as severe.

Both Gail's parents ended up with a diagnosis of dementia, albeit different forms. Her story exemplifies the difficulties family members can face in the lead up to receiving a diagnosis.

Gail's mum's story

Prior to her diagnosis, mum had for some time displayed all the traits of a person living with dementia. She was forgetful, agitated, had mood changes and sometimes showed paranoia. Mum would put items in places they shouldn't be – cleaning products in the fridge, meat in the cupboard and she forgot how to apply her immaculate make-up, a task she had done everyday for over 70 years. But to her there was nothing wrong and she would fly into a rage at the merest hint that she should seek medical advice. At this time I was working full time, and whilst at work one day, I received a call that would change everything – mum had set fire to the house. It wasn't a deliberate act – she had placed a towel over a heater and this then caught fire, causing significant damage to the heater and immediate area around it. Fortunately, my dad managed to extinguish the blaze before it took hold, and thankfully they were both unhurt. However, mum was blissfully unaware of her actions and had no recollection of the incident. This was September 2010.

The following day I spoke with an advanced nurse practitioner at my local GP surgery. I explained everything and she agreed that mum was displaying all the key signs of dementia, but would need to be assessed by her or the GP to get mum into 'the system'. Caroline, the nurse, devised a plan worthy of MI5 to entice mum into the surgery. She gave me a letter explaining that the medical records were being updated for a new system and that the surgery did not have my mum's height or weight. The letter went on to ask if she could call into the surgery for a few minutes so that this could be rectified. Mum fell for it! At last the beginning of our dementia diagnosis was in sight, but for me the panic and fear started to set in having realised just how unprepared I was. Mum was later diagnosed with dementia with Lewy bodies.

Gail's Dad's story

Dad had a stroke in 2002. Fortunately, he made a full recovery within quite a short time. However, we were not made aware at this time that the area of dad's brain that had been significantly affected was the cortex, and that there was a heightened risk that he could develop vascular dementia. The symptoms dad displayed were very subtle, and due to this they were not immediately noticed. He was a little forgetful, but I put this down to his age as the forgetfulness wasn't as extreme as mum's. He also had more mobility problems, but again I thought age and arthritis were responsible.

My mum had an assigned community psychiatric nurse (CPN) who during one of their visits noticed dad's forgetfulness. The CPN took me to one side and suggested that dad should be tested for dementia. At this point I thought 'no, this cannot be happening again'.

An appointment was made with the GP who conducted a simple memory test on dad, which he actually passed. Due to this, the GP stated that there was nothing to worry about and that what the CPN had noticed was due to age.

I wasn't happy with what the GP determined so I spoke with the CPN. He said that he had significant concerns and that dad should be seen by the memory assessment team, and that we should not delay. The CPN spoke with the GP who decided to wait six weeks before calling dad back in to have the simple memory test again. It was at this point he had to agree with the CPN, as dad failed the test on multiple counts. Dad was diagnosed with mixed cortex, subcortical vascular dementia in May 2015.

Gail has provided support and care for both her parents and continues to be the primary care support for her dad, Ron. But these early experiences of wondering what is happening to the person and who to approach for guidance and support are commonly reported difficulties in the research literature (e.g. Innes et al., 2005) that shape people's views and subsequent experiences of dementia care and support.

This pre-diagnosis period can be distressing for all involved as the individual and their family, friends and co-workers recognise a change and seek an explanation. It is common to wonder 'What should I do?' if you are experiencing problems yourself or observing these in your friends or members of your family. These are our recommendations for you to consider if you are worried and no diagnosis has yet been made:

1   Talk to your family doctor.
2   Look for information in your local community and see what support may be available.
3   Do not dismiss your concerns as 'just old age'.
4   Contact the Alzheimer's Society or equivalent voluntary sector organisation.
5   Talk to a trusted relative or friend.
6   Contact any specialist services in your area, for example admiral nurses.

Early diagnosis of dementia can lead to the person being able to live independently for longer and can help to improve quality of life. Receiving help and support sooner can boost confidence both for the person living with dementia and also for the care provider, especially when planning for the future. This planning could include writing a will, financial planning, applying for benefit entitlements and consideration of power of attorney. Support can also be provided by third-sector organisations, day centres, advocacy services, respite care and therapy groups. Access to occupational therapists and mental health support services are also important. The sooner you seek help for any concerns you may have, the quicker you can be assessed and if necessary given a diagnosis and subsequent support and care, for example given medication if appropriate and referred to any local services who may be able to provide practical support to help you adapt. We turn to diagnosis in chapter 2, next.

REFERENCES

Alzheimer Disease International (2012) *World Alzheimer Report 2012 Overcoming the Stigma of Dementia*. www.alz.co.uk/research/World AlzheimerReport2012.pdf

Alzheimer Disease International (2017) *National Dementia Action Plans: Examples For Inspiration*. Swiss Federal Office of Public Health. www. alz.co.uk/sites/default/files/pdfs/national-plans-examples-2017.pdf

Alzheimer Society (n.d.) *Symptoms of Dementia*. www.alzheimers. org.uk/about-dementia/types-dementia/symptoms-dementia [accessed 30 September 2019].

Chertkow, H., Feldman, H.H., Jacova, C. and Massoud, F. (2013) Definitions of dementia and predementia states in Alzheimer's disease and vascular cognitive impairment: Consensus from the Canadian conference on diagnosis of dementia. *Alzheimer's Research & Therapy* 5:S2.

Clark, C., Chaston, D. and Grant, G. (2003) Early interventions in dementia: Carer-led evaluations. In Nolan, M., Lundh, U., Grant, G. and Keady, J. (Eds.), *Partnerships in Family Care: Understanding the Caregiving Career*. Buckingham: University Press.

Department of Health (2012) *Prime Minister's Challenge on Dementia*. London. https://assets.publishing.service.gov.uk/government/uploads/system/uploads/attachment_data/file/215101/dh_133176.pdf

Department of Health (2016) *Challenge on Dementia 2020: Implementation Plan*. https://assets.publishing.service.gov.uk/government/uploads/system/uploads/attachment_data/file/507981/PM_Dementia-main_acc.pdf

Giezendanner, S., Monsch, A.U., Kressig, R.W., Mueller, Y., Streit, S., Essig, S., Zeller, A. and Bally, K. (2019) General practitioners' attitudes towards early diagnosis of dementia: A cross-sectional survey. *BMC Family Practice* 20:65. doi: 10.1186/s12875-019-0956-1

Hackett, R.A., Steptoe, A., Cadar, D. and Fancourt, D. (2019) Social engagement before and after dementia diagnosis in the English Longitudinal Study of Ageing. *PLoS One* 14(8):e0220195. https://doi.org/10.1371/journal.pone.0220195

Illiffe, S. (2015) Evidence-based medicine and dementia. *British Journal of General Practice* 65(639):511–512. https://doi.org/10.3399/bjgp15X686833

Innes, A., Blackstock, K., Mason, A., Smith, A. and Cox, S. (2005) Dementia care provision in rural Scotland: Service users' and carers experiences. *Health and Social Care in the Community* 13(4):354–365.

Jackson, D. (2010) The most difficult decision of my life. In Whitman, L. (Ed.), Telling Tales about Dementia: Experiences of Caring. London: Jessica Kingsley Publishers.

Kim, S., Werner, P., Richardson, A. and Anstey, K.J. (2019) Dementia Stigma Reduction (DESeRvE): Study protocol for a randomized controlled trial of an online intervention program to reduce dementia-related public stigma. *Contemporary Clinical Trials Communications* 14:100351. doi: 10.1016/j.conctc.2019.100351

Le Couteur, D.G., Doust, J., Creasey, H. and Brayne, C. (2013) Political drive to screen for pre-dementia: Not evidence based and ignores the harms of diagnosis. *BMJ* 347. https://doi.org/10.1136/bmj.f5125

Lilford, P. and Hughes, J.C. (2018) Biomarkers and the diagnosis of preclinical dementia. *BJA*. https://doi.org/10.1192/bja.2018.28

Leung, K.K., Finlay, J., Silvius, J.L., Koehn, S., McCleary, L., Cohen, C.A., Hum, S., Garcia, L., Dalziel, W., Emerson, V.F., Pimlott, N.J., Persaud, M., Kozak, J. and Drummond, N. (2011) Pathways to diagnosis: Exploring the experiences of problem recognition and obtaining a dementia diagnosis among Anglo-Canadians. *Health and Social Care in the Community* 19(4):372–381. doi: 10.1111/j.1365-2524.2010.00982.x. Epub 2011 January 11.

McCleary, L., Persaud, M., Hum, S., Pimlott, N.J., Cohen, C.A., Koehn, S., Leung, K.K., Dalziel, W.B., Kozak, J., Emerson, V.F., Silvius, J.L., Garcia, L. and Drummond, N. (2013) Pathways to dementia diagnosis among South Asian Canadians. *Dementia* 12(6):769–789. doi: 10.1177/1471301212444806

National Audit Office (2007) *Improving Services and Support for People with Dementia.* London: Stationary Office. www.nao.org.uk/publications/nao_reports/06-07/0607604.pdf

Palmer, K., Bäckman, L., Winblad, B. and Fratiglioni, L. (2003) Detection of Alzheimer's disease and dementia in the preclinical phase: Population based cohort study. *BMJ* 326(7383):245.

Perry-Young, L., Owen, G., Kelly, S. and Owens, C. (2018) How people come to recognise a problem and seek medical help for a person showing early signs of dementia: A systematic review and meta-ethnography. *Dementia* 17(1):34–60.

Prince, M., Comas-Herrera, A., Knapp, M., Guerchet, M. and Kara-giannidou, M. (2016) *World Alzheimer Report 2016: Improving Healthcare for People Living with Dementia: Coverage, Quality and Costs Now and in the Future.* London, UK: Alzheimer's Disease International (ADI).

Robinson, H. (2010) Glimpses of glory on a long, grey road. In Whitman, L. (Ed.), Telling Tales about Dementia: Experiences of Caring. London: Jessica Kingsley Publishers.

Steeman, E., De Casterles, B.D., Godderis, J. and Grypdonck, M. (2006) Living with early-stage dementia: A review of qualitative studies. Journal of Advanced Nursing 54(6):722–738.

Woods, R., Moniz-Cook, E., Iliffe, S., Campion, P., Vernooij-Dassen, M., Zanetti, O. and Franco, M. (2003) Dementia: Issues in early recognition and intervention in primary care. *Journal of the Royal Society of Medicine* 96:320–324.

2

DIAGNOSIS OF DEMENTIA

There have been many developments since the turn of the twenty-first century when the issue of diagnosis of dementia began to be hotly debated. Common questions that have been explored by clinicians, policy makers, researchers and people living with dementia and their families are:

- How can the diagnosis be given more quickly, or in a more timely manner?
- Who should give the diagnosis?
- Why have there been difficulties in giving the diagnosis?
- How can professionals improve their skills in giving the diagnosis to the person with dementia?
- What can be done to improve the diagnostic experience for the person with the condition and their family?

Importantly, these are issues that people living with dementia and their families have raised (e.g. Laron et al., 2018). Diagnosis of many conditions is a complex process, and this is also the case for dementia. Understanding the diagnosis as part of a process and not as a single event is important. It also needs to be contextualised from the viewpoint of both the person who is diagnosed as having a dementia and their family, but also from the viewpoint of the many health practitioners who are involved. In their review, Koch and Iliffe (2010) suggest a variety of factors influencing the diagnostic process. They group these factors into three primary types that contribute to delays in an individual receiving the diagnosis: patient factors, GP factors and system characteristics.

As we noted in our pre-diagnosis discussion in chapter 1, the person experiencing concerns in their functioning and abilities and/or their family members may delay getting advice due to a lack of knowledge about the symptoms of dementia, fear of stigma or due to them misattributing the areas of concern to old age. These would all fall under what Koch and Iliffe (2010) have called 'patient factors'. Government policies have specifically attempted to address lack of knowledge and awareness in the UK (Department of Health, 2012) and internationally (Alzheimer Disease International, 2017) and this reflects the World Health Organisation's call (2012) for dementia to be a global health priority. Yet, Iliffe and Manthorpe (2004) raised the question of hazards of the early recognition of dementia: the demand for assessment based upon the "Alzheimerisation" of older age, demand to meet the needs of those traumatised by the diagnosis and the resource pressure of supporting more people for longer, a view upheld by others (Pratt et al., 2006). An earlier or more timely diagnosis will not necessarily 'fix' the issues that have been recognised as problematic.

EARLY DIAGNOSIS AND TIMELY DIAGNOSIS

Diagnosis has long been perceived as a key part of the assessment of a person with dementia by many practitioners (Jacques and Jackson, 2000) with the pros and cons of an early diagnosis debated (Fox et al., 2013). The early diagnosis of dementia has been supported by policy directives (World Health Organisation, 2012; Alzheimer Disease International, 2017) because it helps people to understand what is happening to them, access support and services and plan ahead. Increasingly, in the UK, the focus is on the GP and the wider primary care team as the most appropriate professionals to identify people who may be experiencing cognitive impairment and to make the initial diagnosis.

The pre-diagnostic processes that lead to the point of diagnosis can take some time. For some individuals this may be relatively quick, but for others it can take a few years (e.g. Innes et al., 2005; Parker et al., 2020). Another indication of time to the point of diagnosis is from research where people with dementia have been found to have visited their GP more often than others in the two years prior to diagnosis (Bamford et al., 2007), indicating the length of time that individuals and their families live with concerns before receiving a diagnosis. In Australia, Speechly et al. (2009) found that symptoms of dementia for their 415-person sample had been present 1.9 years before approaching a health professional and that a diagnosis took 3.1 years after first being concerned with symptoms. In one area of the UK the average time for participants in the study to have noticed there may be a problem to receiving a full diagnosis was 3 years (Chrisp et al., 2011) with delays at three points accounting for these time lags: first in noticing there is a problem, second in talking to someone to share concerns that there may be a problem with a health care professional and then a third period of delay when the health care system has been alerted to these concerns.

There are differences in who receives a diagnosis and how quickly. This can vary significantly depending on where one lives, for example, in remote and rural locations (Innes et al., 2011) and on individuals' background characteristics, for example, ethnicity (McCleary et al., 2012). Most tests to help diagnose dementia, such as the Mini-Mental State Examination (MMSE) are developed in a colour-blind manner. This leads to inaccurate diagnosis and misunderstandings (Rait, 2000). In the UK and Ireland there are three main indigenous minority languages: Welsh, Scottish Gaelic and Irish Gaelic. It is generally held that those whose first language is not English will lose their fluency of English as their cognitive impairment increases. In the Morgan and Crowder (2003) small-scale study of Welsh speakers and the MMSE:

42 percent scored better in Welsh
19 percent had consistent scores in both languages
39 percent performed better in English

These findings support the view that language alone can alter someone's performance rating. They go on to observe:

In the context that decisions about the allocation of health and social care services are increasingly made on the basis of people's scores on

a screening instrument, this may have potentially significant consequences, both for those concerned whose ability to live independently
may be questioned and also for the health and social care services
where resources may be inappropriately targeted.

(Morgan and Crowder, 2003, 271)

Rait et al. (2000) highlight that culture and ethnicity also impact on
the accuracy of a screening instrument. Rait et al. (2000) worked
to adapt the MMSE and the Abbreviated Mental Test (AMT) into
five languages commonly used by older South Asians in Britain.
The findings were encouraging in that the modified screening tests
were acceptable to the people they were administered to and offered
a more accurate measurement of cognitive impairment. The tools
were adapted through a lengthy process involving three working
groups: academics, translators and South Asian people. Some questions and their wording were changed to achieve the desired measure. For example, the date of the First World War was changed to the
date of Independence. This study underlines the need to broaden the
range of tools to take account of race and culture.

Despite these early recognitions of the need for cultural sensitivity, recent work in Norway has found that GPs struggle to assess
and diagnose dementia with immigrant populations due to language
barriers and reliance on family members to interpret, as well as a lack
of knowledge of culturally appropriate assessment tools (Sagbakken
et al., 2018). A recent review of studies of South Asians experiences
of dementia (Blakemore et al., 2018) reveals the continued lack of
validated, culturally appropriate diagnostic tools that may then lead
to a diagnosis and access to appropriate services.

Culture and ethnicity are only two of many factors that can impact
on the diagnosis, as demonstrated by US research where a whole range
of factors were found to influence diagnosis. Amjad et al. (2017) found
that males, younger participants, non-whites and those with less than
a high school education were less likely to be diagnosed. They also
found that those who went to medical appointments alone, who could
manage their own medications and who could still manage everyday
living were less likely to be diagnosed. These variations in experiences
of diagnosis have contributed to the calls for earlier diagnosis, but in
turn have led to debates on a 'timely' diagnosis (Robinson et al., 2015),
as earlier is not always seen to be better for the person with dementia

or their families (Rimmer, 2016).Yet as has been clearly stated, the rate of undiagnosed people clearly places an imperative on an approach that will achieve the best outcomes for people living with dementia and their families (Burns et al., 2014).

When and how to give the diagnosis has received much attention from health care professionals. Around a decade ago targets were developed in the UK to increase the rates of diagnosis of dementia (Scottish Government, 2008; Department of Health, 2009), as it was recognised that the rates of disclosure were significantly lower than that of cancer (Bamford et al., 2004). It has been found that understandings of dementia have shaped UK dementia policies and influenced the types of initiatives that receive government support (Innes and Manthorpe, 2013). Policies reflect that dementia is understood to be a health condition but over time there has been an increased recognition that raising awareness of dementia within society (Department of Health, 2012, 2016) and promoting a supportive environment may lead to people being able to live well with dementia, and relatively independently, for longer.

Thus, although rates of diagnosis have improved rapidly there is still variability in the rates of diagnosis within countries (Walker et al., 2017), the experiences of receiving a diagnosis have not always improved (Watson et al., 2018) and the outcomes for families and people living with dementia are variable (Woods et al., 2019). Policy directives have increasingly shaped the drive to increase the numbers of people with dementia receiving a diagnosis, as it has been recognised that this is the gateway to receiving support and management (Donegan et al., 2017). In a clinical review Robinson et al. (2015) discuss the case for a *timely diagnosis* and early intervention while noting that there are many factors that health care professionals will take into account when deciding when to refer, when to give the diagnosis and the way they think is best to share the diagnosis and provide signposting to further support. There is a genuine complexity surrounding the diagnosis of dementia given that it is an umbrella term for many different symptoms with underlying causes. The need for a timely diagnosis is something that has been stressed by many people living with dementia involved in research studies across the globe (Watson et al., 2018; Laron et al., 2018). There has therefore been a move in discussion from early detection to a 'timely' diagnosis, and researchers have been concerned as to what this means for clinicians (Robinson et al., 2015; Dhedhi et al., 2014; Manthorpe et al., 2013), the person living with dementia (Watson et al., 2018) and their families (Woods et al., 2019).

WHO SHOULD GIVE THE DIAGNOSIS?

There has been lively discussion and debate in the research literature about who should give a diagnosis; what the challenges are in giving a diagnosis; the different perspectives different practitioners have on diagnosis; the different experiences of diagnosis as reported by people living with dementia and their care partners; and how to disclose the diagnosis (van den Dungen et al., 2014; Werner et al., 2013; Bamford et al., 2004). Calls have been made to create pathways to ensure that a single approach is taken to the process of diagnosis.

The role of the general practitioner or family physician

The role of the GP is an area that has received much debate in the last decade. General practitioners, or family physicians, have been seen as the gatekeepers to services because they are most likely to be the professional whom relatives approach for help. Early work in this area (Downs, 1996; Downs et al., 2002a) argued for the potential role of GPs to:

- Identify people who are suspected of having a dementia.
- Exclude treatable causes.
- Refer to specialist psychiatric services when diagnosis is uncertain.
- Provide information about the diagnosis and prognosis.
- Assess the family carers' capacity to continue caring.
- Signpost services and welfare benefits.
- Help with access to services.
- Provide emotional support to family carers.
- Attend to the wider medical needs of the person with dementia and their carers.

Other research into GPs and early diagnosis (Milne et al., 2000) both confirmed and challenged the above, finding:

- Ambivalence towards the value of early diagnosis.
- Reluctance to extend work into a difficult and demanding area.
- Improvement in services is not a strong motivator to encourage early intervention.

Other early research highlighted GPs' failure to follow through recommended procedures such as screening for other causes of confusion and for depression (Downs et al., 2002a; Fortinsky, 2000). Also there was a noted discrepancy between what doctors said they offered to people with dementia and their carers and what the carers stated they were offered (Maslow et al., 2002).

Reports from the early 2000s consistently suggested that GPs knew little about dementia, lack the skills to identify it and are not supported to manage it (National Audit Office, 2007; Audit Commission, 2000). Downs et al. (2006) collected the views of the carers of people with dementia on the responses of GPs when they were first approached about the person with dementia. The findings from this study suggest that, overall, carers felt they got a 'good' service from their GPs. On closer examination, however, the picture was more complex; even when carers expressed satisfaction with their GP this did not necessarily mean they had received a satisfactory service. GPs with good inter-personal skills, for example, those who were good at listening and responding to stated needs and concerns were valued by carers (Downs et al., 2006). An Australian study found that GPs did not always feel there was a benefit to giving a diagnosis (Hansen et al., 2008) for a myriad of reasons and that they were reluctant to provide a diagnosis if they felt that it would not positively impact on the persons' life. In a study evaluating feasibility of screening for and diagnosing dementia in a rural population in the US, Boise et al. (2010) identified that, with training in the use of screening instruments, the rate of screening and diagnosing dementia increased. Of particular importance is the fact that confidence of clinicians increased during the study. Recipients of the screening programme also reported satisfaction with the process. This study highlights the value of workplace training to aid the diagnostic process.

More recent research highlights that GPs have improved in the rates of their diagnosing dementia but that the rates vary across different geographical locations within a country (Walker et al., 2017). Reasons for these variances are similar to the issues first raised in the early 2000s. For example, Phillips et al.'s (2012) study of GPs in Australia found that GPs reported a lack of confidence in having a correct diagnosis, that they were concerned to act in patients' best interests and that the stigma associated with the 'dementia' label influenced their disclosure process.

Doctors in memory clinics in the UK understood the importance of naming dementia and the delicacy required when being honest but not letting go of hope when discussing prognosis and medication (Bailey et al., 2018). However, this is a difficult balance in the absence of high-quality support services being available to refer on to following the diagnosis.

In a recent study of how GPs communicate the diagnosis of dementia, Dooley et al. (2018) found that all GPs named dementia directly when giving the diagnosis, but that they used different strategies to talk about prognosis. This demonstrates a sensitivity and awareness of the need for individuals and their families to process what dementia might mean for them. In the US, Zaleta et al. (2010) examined the use of person-centred communication when delivering a diagnosis and found that individual physicians were consistent in their approach but that there was variance between the person-centredness of different physicians. The impact this had on the recipient of the diagnosis was not investigated but is clearly an area that would warrant further investigation, to determine whether the approach of the diagnoser has an impact on the diagnosee.

Overall, research has shown that GPs can find it challenging to identify dementia in the consultation context and that they would prefer to disclose the diagnosis when a family member is also present. GPs use different communication strategies to share the diagnosis and may try to soften the message by using euphemisms and trying to offer hope.

Wider primary care team input

The emphasis on the wider primary care team has been developed within national dementia strategies and plans. Community and practice nurses may be asked to visit someone for another nursing task but this person may also present with early symptoms of dementia. As such they are well placed to identify the need for further assessment. This might include pain assessment, review of medication or referral to a continence nurse. Manthorpe et al.'s (2003) survey of community mental health, community and practice nurses exploring their ability and confidence in diagnosing and supporting people in giving a diagnosis of dementia found that, generally, nurses agreed on the possible early symptoms of dementia. Mental health nurses had more confidence and knowledge about how to assess and support the person, although some of the other nurses were already engaging in the diagnostic process and referral on to relevant services. As a result, researchers argue that this role for nurses in general should be developed through training. Also, informal good practices which encourage involvement of the wider primary care team should be formalised without an overemphasis on the ideal care pathway. Early work in this area revealed a need for an educational strategy for primary care (Downs et al., 2002a; Iliffe et al., 2003; Turner et al., 2003; DoH, 2009) and has contributed to the policy drivers in the UK and internationally (Alzheimer Disease International, 2017) to detect dementia earlier and to provide a timely diagnosis.

Care pathways

The need for a coordinated approach to provide services for people with dementia and their care partners has been argued to be crucial (Department of Health, 2012). Care pathways have developed to try to ensure a smooth passage between diagnosis and subsequent services for the person with dementia. In addition, there has been a recognition of the need to improve the practice of identifying and then diagnosing dementia as a part of the process of supporting people with dementia and their families (Alzheimer Disease International, 2017).

There can be a presumption that diagnosis will be a stepping stone to relevant help and support for the person with dementia and those who provide support, yet members of the British Medical Association have expressed strong concerns that this is not actually the case (Rimmer, 2016). Care pathways have been developed, originating from the NHS but incorporating other services to improve the access, experience and coordination of the services people receive. Care pathways should be based upon an agreed protocol of the relevant agencies.

A care pathway aims to ensure that connections are made between:

- the right people
- doing the right things
- in the right order
- at the right time
- in the right place
- with the right outcome
- all with attention to the patient experience

In this way care pathways may level the playing field for individuals undergoing diagnosis in any area of the country as the same processes would be followed no matter where a person lives.

Upskilling, education and training

Research has revealed how we can begin to find realistic ways to enable practitioners to diagnose better. Education and training is one way of doing this. In particular, the push for primary care practitioners to be more involved in diagnosis continues to need careful thought. GPs may be well placed in terms of being more accessible to the person and their family but the nature of their workload and traditional practices may hamper their confidence and abilities to diagnose (Phillips et al., 2012). The wider primary health care staff may be particularly well placed to broaden their role in the process leading up to a diagnosis with people with dementia. The establishment of memory clinics does not necessarily reduce this role because they are a specialist, time-limited resource for primary care teams and access to these is therefore limited. The first point of health care contact may continue to be the GP or district nursing services.

Educational programmes for psychiatrists have been developed (Robinson et al., 2010) and other research has argued for the need for more training and education to support doctors in giving the diagnosis; for example it has been argued that doctors in memory clinics would benefit from evidence-based training and supervision to prepare them for these emotionally challenging and complex consultations where a diagnosis is given (Bailey et al., 2018) and that training to help GPs recognise the benefits to people with dementia and their families of receiving a diagnosis (Hansen et al., 2008) is also required.

DISCLOSING THE DIAGNOSIS: THE EXPERIENCE OF PEOPLE LIVING WITH DEMENTIA AND THEIR FAMILY MEMBERS

Disclosing to the person with dementia their diagnosis is an area fraught with conflicting views and opinions. Clearly, a pivotal motivation must also be informing the person and their family of the diagnosis and giving them information and ongoing support as they start to register and react to the diagnosis. Pratt and Wilkinson (2003) developed a model of understanding people's responses to diagnosis, based on their research into this issue. However, Downs et al.'s (2002b) survey of GPs revealed that the nature of the information provided varied considerably.

For example, research has demonstrated that even when the care partner themselves would want a diagnosis if they had dementia, they have reservations about the diagnosis being given to their relative (Bamford et al., 2004). Bamford et al. (2004) found that professionals often disclose to the carer rather than the person with dementia and may separate individuals to give the diagnosis. Milne (2000) research into GPs and early diagnosis highlight:

- Ambivalence towards the value of early diagnosis.
- Reluctance to extend work into a difficult and demanding area.
- Improvement in services not being a strong motivator to encourage early intervention.

Professionals who do disclose the diagnosis often differ in the terms they use; some use specific terms like Alzheimer's disease while others prefer terms such as confusion. Many also find it difficult to give the diagnosis and find it to be a more time-consuming process than giving a diagnosis of other conditions. Connell et al. (2009) identified that family members reported benefits to diagnosis including obtaining information, having an explanation for the changes noted and prompting future plans; these findings should reassure GPs that a diagnosis can be a useful process for families. However, Connell et al. (2009) also reported barriers to diagnosis including lack of a cure, the perception that nothing could be done for the person and lack of an effective treatment, indicating that more work needs to be done to change perceptions of dementia.

Xanthopoulou et al. (2019) found that when disclosing the diagnosis many concerns are raised by the person living with dementia and their care companions. This demonstrates the need to give time to the diagnostic delivery and to answer the concerns that individuals and their care companions may have.

In Canada, participants who had received a diagnosis of dementia demonstrated three forms of response categorised by the researchers (Aminzadeh et al., 2007) as (1) responses suggesting a denial or lack of insight into the diagnosis, (2) grief reactions related to the experience of actual or anticipated losses and (3) positive coping responses to maximise what this might mean for their lives.

Few of Mathorpe et al.'s (2013) UK participants found the process of memory assessment to be patient centred. Assessment processes were experienced as lengthy and for some distressing and conducted in settings that participants found alarming or stigmatising. They also found that communication and sharing of information was variable and practitioners were not always thought to help people to make sense of their experiences.

Different groups of people with dementia and their carers therefore have different experiences of diagnosis. For example, younger people with dementia often face greater delays to diagnosis and the process is complicated by factors such as lack of understanding and awareness. Understanding the issues for different groups can help to improve understanding of the diagnostic process for all people with dementia, and these will now be briefly explored.

Diagnosis for people from black and minority ethnic (BAME) groups can be particularly difficult. La Fontaine et al. (2007) found little recognition or understanding of the term dementia among a group of British South Asians of all ages. Dementia was seldom mentioned in discussions of ageing and ageing-associated difficulties. Ageing was seen as a time of withdrawal and isolation. There was the suggestion amongst this group that the symptoms of dementia may result from 'lack of effort from the person themselves and possibly from a lack of family care' (La Fontaine et al., 2007, 605). This lack of understanding suggests that there is a gap in knowledge amongst this community which needs to be addressed by primary health care and other services as attitudes held by groups are likely to lead to delays in diagnosis. Canadian research exploring the experiences of Canadian Asians also found that a delay in diagnosis could be linked to families' cultural understandings of ageing and also their lack of knowledge about dementia and a tendency to explain problems in relation to ageing and personality (McCleary et al., 2012).

Demographic information such as age, medical or psychiatric diagnosis provides only a partial view of a person's situation. The person also needs to be considered in relation to their family and wider environment. There is a need to discover the person's strengths and abilities and perceptions of their lives. How the person is experiencing the illness and how they are trying to compensate for it also needs to be considered. Equally families will react in both practical and emotional ways to the person with dementia (Aminzadeh et al.,

2007; Cahill et al., 2008; Bunn et al., 2012). An explicit framework supported by knowledge and research is essential to ensure that the experience of diagnosis is as constructive as possible to the person and their family. Often though, practitioners make shortcuts based on incomplete information due to past experiences of similar situations, pressure of time or preconceptions of the 'problem'. There is a tendency to work in boxes: hospital ward, memory clinic, home care, health centre, care home and community care team, for example. However, people's care and support needs do not fit into the neat service boxes and an individual may need the support of all these services (and others) at different moments in time.

There is as yet little evidence of a widespread change in the diagnostic services people with dementia receive, but there is considerable interest and debate into how to improve things. But the experiences of two of this book's authors demonstrate the difficulties in the diagnostic experiences.

Gerry Bowker's story as experienced by her daughter Gail

In 2010 my beautiful mum, Gerry, was diagnosed with dementia with Lewy bodies. I can remember the day vividly, but for all the wrong reasons.

Pre-dementia, mum had always been wary of doctors and hospitals. Luckily she had been blessed with good health, having been in hospital only twice in her life – one of those being to give birth to me! As a result, I actually dreaded the moment of having to take her to the memory assessment clinic. As we left our house I told my mum that we were going for a short drive – all was well until we approached the gates of the clinic and she saw the words WOODLANDS HOSPITAL. Mum became distressed, screaming and crying almost like a young child. At this point I was struggling with my own emotions and just wanted to wrap her in a cotton wool blanket and take her back home. But I knew we had to proceed. Dad came too, and I could see how distressed he was at seeing the love of his life so terrified that she was trembling as we entered through the doors.

Once inside, mum started to calm down a little, as the reception was far from looking like a hospital. The receptionist was kind and offered mum a drink of tea, as she could see that mum was upset. However, that was only a short respite. We were ushered into a room that had a table, chairs, no windows and nothing on the walls. A kind-looking nurse came into the room, took some details and then asked mum to go with her into another room. Mum was reluctant and kept looking at dad and I for reassurance. For two hours we were separated from mum. Dad and I were being asked questions relating to mum's behaviours and memory, whilst mum was being assessed. The nurse with dad and I said that it wasn't usual for the testing to take so long, and she would find out what the issue was. Eventually mum came back into the room, and I was asked to follow the nurse who had conducted the assessment. I was told that mum had struggled with almost every part of the test, and that she was showing signs of distress and agitation. I explained that this was because mum was afraid of hospitals and that I should have been allowed to be with her.

I was taken into a separate room where the consultant quietly gave me the diagnosis, then further explained that no treatment would be offered as mum was already classified as 'too severe' due to only scoring 12/100 on her Addenbrooke's Cognitive Examination (ACE). I was handed a photocopied piece of paper which gave a pressé of dementia. I was then told that the centre was closing at 5 p.m. prompt, so if I had any questions could I pose them. This was at 4:45 p.m. – 15 minutes to process what I had just been told and to form questions there and then. My head was in a whir and yes I did have questions – lots of them, but had no idea where to start. I was angry at the way the meeting was going and felt somehow let down by the process, so asked to meet with the doctor at a time more convenient. She sighed, then agreed to meet the following week.

Mum only scored 12/100, which meant she was diagnosed as severe. I believed this test was not a true reflection of mum's cognitive ability. I felt that had she been tested at our home, as is allowed now, the outcome would have been very different. From 2010 until 2017 her cognitive ability varied very little. She could still follow conversations, had reasoning ability, could still carry out mathematical equations and still recognised dad and me. Having been given a severe diagnosis so early on in her dementia had a knock-on effect later. It meant that she was declined cancer treatment in the last 18 months of her life, she was not offered anti-dementia drugs and she was virtually written off by a number of professionals.

Unfortunately Gail's father then experienced symptoms leading to a diagnosis of dementia.

Ron Bowker's story as told by his daughter Gail

Dad was diagnosed with mixed cortex, subcortical vascular dementia in 2015. As a family we had already lived with dementia for five years, so when dad received his diagnosis I wasn't as shocked or fazed. Having experience of the way the system worked was a massive help, as I knew who to contact and where to get information and support from. Thankfully there had been significant improvements in the post-diagnostic support – though there were gaps, it was certainly better than when mum was diagnosed.

The Addenbrookes Cognitive Examination (ACE) was conducted at our home, which was an improvement on my mum's experience, allowing for dad to be more relaxed in surroundings he was comfortable with. The only issue was that dad also has sight impairment, and the test relied on dad being able to draw a clock face and to identify objects – which as you can imagine proved extremely difficult. Due to this he didn't score as well as I had expected he would.

Dad was later invited to have a brain scan, and I was surprisingly allowed to be present with him. This was a change from when my mum had hers as I was not allowed to even walk down the corridor with her – which was distressing for mum and I in equal measures, so much so that her scan had to be cancelled.

Even though the process of diagnosis had improved from when mum was diagnosed, there were still gaps and areas for enhancement. Following dad's initial diagnosis I was originally told that dad had mixed dementia. However, several months later, and following a conversation I had with a consultant, I was told that dad had been wrongly diagnosed. He actually had mixed cortex, subcortical vascular dementia. This was a result of a stroke he suffered in 2002. I asked why there had been an error in the diagnosis and was told that it is common to wrongly diagnose dementia in the early stages of the disease. Naturally I was quite annoyed at this point as I had been given slight hope that dad would be started on Aricept – an anti-dementia drug. However this was quickly 'shot down in flames' as vascular dementia has no magic pill – there is no cure.

Lesley's account of the diagnostic process as a person going through the diagnosis demonstrates the fear, awareness of stigma and then the pressing need to try and do something to alleviate the symptoms and make life as bearable as possible.

Lesley's story

The doctor referred me to the memory clinic at the Woodlands where I attended with my husband. I cancelled the first appointment because I was embarrassed (mental health has a stigma). I thought I might bump into one of my patients, and I also convinced myself there was nothing wrong and I was wasting their time.

Everyone at the Woodlands made me feel at ease. I saw the consultant and had a memory test which I thought went OK, but I didn't score as high as I should have. I was then referred for an MRI scan. The consultant suggested I take time off work but I didn't want to, I wasn't ill. I carried on working and at the end of February when things got worse and I was forgetting more important things, I decided to take the doctors' advice.

When the results of the MRI scan came back I was referred to the Cerebral Function Unit at Salford Royal Hospital, as the scan showed enlarged ventricles, and this could have been causing the memory loss. However, after more memory psychological and neurological tests I was seen by the doctor and then a social worker and told I was unable to return to work at all.

Whilst this was going on, I had signed up for a drug trial on a new drug for Alzheimer's in Warrington. After numerous memory tests, blood tests, lumber puncture and MRI tests, I was told because of the enlarged ventricles I was not able to continue in the trial. They have strict criteria for drug trials. However, the consultant was so concerned about the results of all the tests that he had collected he rang me and said he was sending them to the Woodlands, because if I was his patient he would put me on medication straight away. The medication is not a cure but it slows down the condition. So although I didn't make it to the end of the drug trial, it did actually help.

Returning to the Woodlands to see the psychiatrist, I was given a diagnosis of mild Alzheimer's and offered medication. I have never been one for taking medication. However, as I was finding it difficult to remember and communicate, and I knew there was no cure, the only choice was to try the medication.

I think if I was being diagnosed today, I would have taken a pen and paper with me and I would have written questions down that I would have liked to ask, then wrote down the answers that I received, because as soon as you hear the word dementia your brain just closes and you don't hear anything else.

Perhaps it would be a good idea if you could be given the name of somebody living with dementia who could give you some personal tips, such as places to go for financial advice or groups to keep you from becoming a recluse. You are more likely to become a recluse if you have dementia and live alone.

Being given a stack of papers such as how the medication works, power of attorney and type of dementia is not the ideal way to be given this diagnosis. It would be better if there was somebody who had the time to explain it slowly and thoroughly to you, including where to go and get help, how to keep connected and prevent you getting depressed.

I know those giving the diagnosis would probably like to do this, but the doctors and nurses don't have enough time, and there is not enough money in the National Health Service. However, I feel if more time is given at diagnosis this would help you accept the diagnosis and you would feel more positive about it all.

Research evidence and the experiences of people living with dementia and their families provides us with ideas about what might be helpful to bear in mind if going through the diagnosis as an individual or as a family member.

Tips for the person and their family undergoing the diagnosis process

1   Ask to have a family member/friend present as you will not digest everything. Being told that you have dementia can be traumatic. Support is what you need at those initial stages.

2   If you are unsure of what has been said, ask for everything in writing.

3   Make sure that you are offered support. You may not think that you need it at first, but as the news sinks in and you have time to reflect, you will find having professional support in the guise of a CPN or dementia support worker is crucial.

4   If you are uncomfortable with 'hospital' environments, ask to take the memory test in a place you feel comfortable.

5   If you have any sensory impairment, ensure that the assessment centre are aware of this. Adaptations can be made.
6   Make sure that the test is carried out in your first language.
7   Make sure that you make professionals aware of any concerns you have, and if you feel overwhelmed, ask to stop.

The point of diagnosis is critical not only for the person and their family but also for the services they might require in the future. Therefore, when we look at responses and reactions by the person who has been diagnosed and their families and the types of services they might welcome at this point in time, these need to be contextualised in their experiences up to the point of diagnosis. We will look at the efforts to improve ongoing services by the development of care pathways and the idea that diagnosis should open up offers of support and information which makes the person's journey smoother and qualitatively better via post-diagnostic support. The experience leading up to the diagnosis and the diagnosis itself can leave people living with dementia and their families in need of support and further information. In the next section, we turn to *post-diagnostic support*.

REFERENCES

Alzheimer Disease International (2017) *National Dementia Action Plans: Examples for Inspiration.* Swiss Federal Office of Public Health. www.alz.co.uk/sites/default/files/pdfs/national-plans-examples-2017.pdf

Aminzadeh, F., Byszewski, A., Molnar, F.J. and Eisner, M. (2007) Emotional impact of dementia diagnosis: Exploring persons with dementia and caregivers' perspectives. *Aging and Mental Health* 11(3):281–290.

Amjad, H., Ahuja, A., Lyketsos, C., Roth, D.L. and Samus, Q.M. (2017) Patterns in formal dementia diagnosis and awareness of diagnosis. *Alzheimer's and Dementia* 13(7), Supplement, P841. https://doi.org/10.1016/j.jalz.2017.06.1181

Audit Commission (2000) *Forget Me Not: Developing Mental Health Services for Older People in England.* London: Audit Commission.

Bailey, C., Dooley, J. and McCabe, R. (2018) "How do they want to know?" Doctors' perspectives on making and communicating a diagnosis of dementia. *Dementia*. https://doi.org/10.1177/1471301218763904

Bamford, C., Eccles, M., Steen, N. and Robinson, L. (2007) Can primary care record review facilitate earlier diagnosis of dementia? *Family Practice* 24(2):108–116.

Bamford, C., Lamont, S., Eccles, M., Robinson, L., May, C. and Bond, J. (2004) Disclosing a diagnosis of dementia: A systematic review. *International Journal Geriatric Psychiatry* 19(2):151–169.

Blakemore, A., Kenning, C., Mirza, N., Daker-White, G., Panagioti, M. and Waheed, W. (2018) Dementia in UK South Asians: A scoping review of the literature. *BMJ Open* 8:e020290. doi: 10.1136/bmjopen-2017-020290

Boise, L., Eckstrom, E., Fagnan, L., King, A., Goubaud, M., Buckley, D. I. and Morris, C. (2010) The rural older adult memory (ROAM) study: A practice-based intervention to improve dementia screening and diagnosis. *Journal of the American Board of Family Medicine (JABFM)* 23(4):486–498. https://doi.org/10.3122/jabfm.2010.04.090225

Bunn, F., Goodman, C., Sworn, K., Rait, G., Brayne, C., Robinson, L., McNeilly, E. and Iliffe, S. (2012) Psychosocial factors that shape patient and carer experiences of dementia diagnosis and treatment: A systematic review of qualitative studies. *PLOS Medicine* 9(10):e1001331.

Burns, A., Hughes, J. and Rasmussen, J. (2014) Achieving quality of care in dementia by appropriate and timely diagnosis. *BMJ: British Medical Journal* 348:G3199.

Cahill, S.M., Gibb, M., Bruce, I., Headon, M. and Drury, M. (2008) "I was worried coming in because I don't really know why it was arranged": The subjective experience of new patients and their primary caregivers attending a memory clinic. *Dementia* 7(2):175–189.

Chrisp, T.A.C., Thomas, B.D., Goddard, W.A. and Owens, A. (2011) Dementia timeline: Journeys, delays and decisions on the pathway to an early diagnosis. *Dementia* 10(4):555–570.

Connell, C.M., Roberts, J.S., McLaughlin, S.J. and Carpenter, B.D. (2009) Black and white adult family members' attitudes toward a dementia diagnosis. *Journal of the American Geriatrics Society* 57(9):1562–1568.

Department of Health (2009) *Living Well with Dementia: A National Dementia Strategy*. London. https://assets.publishing.service.gov.uk/government/uploads/system/uploads/attachment_data/file/168220/dh_094051.pdf

Department of Health (2012) *Prime Minister's Challenge on Dementia*. London. https://assets.publishing.service.gov.uk/government/uploads/system/uploads/attachment_data/file/215101/dh_133176.pdf

Department of Health (2016) *Challenge on Dementia 2020: Implementation Plan*. https://assets.publishing.service.gov.uk/government/uploads/system/uploads/attachment_data/file/507981/PM_Dementia-main_acc.pdf

Dhedhi, S.A., Swinglehurst, D. and Russell, J. (2014) "Timely" diagnosis of dementia: What does it mean? A narrative analysis of GPs' accounts. *BMJ Open* 4(3):E004439. doi: 10.1136/bmjopen-2013-004439

Donegan, K., Fox, N., Black, N., Livingston, G., Banerjee, S. and Burns, A. (2017) Trends in diagnosis and treatment for people with dementia in the UK from 2005 to 2015: A longitudinal retrospective cohort study. *The Lancet*. https://doi.org/10.1016/S2468-2677(17)30031-2

Dooley, J., Bass, N. and McCabe, R. (2018) How do doctors deliver a diagnosis of dementia in memory clinics? *British Journal of Psychiatry* 212(4):239–245. https://doi.org/10.1192/bjp.2017.64

Downs, M. (1996) The role of general practice in dementia diagnosis and management. *International Journal of Geriatric Psychiatry* 11:937–942.

Downs, M., Ariss, S.M.B., Grant, E., Keady, J., Turner, S., Bryans, M. Wilcokc, J, Levin, E., O'Carroll, R. and Iliffe, S. (2006). Family carers' accounts of general practice contacts for their relatives with early signs of dementia. *Dementia* 5(3):353–373. https://doi.org/10.1177/1471301206067111

Downs, M., Cook, A., Rae, C. and Collins, K.E. (2002a) Caring for patients with dementia: The GP perspective. *Aging and Mental Health* 4(4):301–304.

Downs, M., Clibbens, R., Rae, C., Cook, A. and Woods, R. (2002b) What do general practitioners tell people with dementia and their families about the condition? A survey of experiences in Scotland. *Dementia* 1(1):47–58.

Fortinsky, R.H. (2000) Edititorial: Dementia and depression in older persons: Cross national challenges to primary care medicine. *Aging and Mental Health* 4(4):283–285.

Fox, C., Lafortune, L., Boustani, M. and Brayne, C. (2013) The pros and cons of early diagnosis in dementia. *British Journal General Practice* 63(612):e510–e512.

Hansen, E.C., Hughes, C., Routley, G. and Robinson, A.L. (2008) General practitioners' experiences and understandings of diagnosing dementia: Factors impacting on early diagnosis. *Social Science and Medicine* 67(11):1776–1783.

Iliffe, S. and Manthorpe, J. (2004) The hazards of early recognition of dementia: A risk assessment. *Aging and Mental Health* 8(2):99–105.

Iliffe, S., Manthorpe, J. and Eden, A. (2003) Sooner or later? Issues in the early diagnosis of dementia in general practice: A qualitative study. *Family Practice* 20(4):376–381. doi.org/10.1093/fampra/cmg407

Innes, A., Blackstock, K., Mason, A., Smith, A. and Cox, S. (2005) Dementia care provision in rural Scotland: Service users' and carers experiences. *Health and Social Care in the Community* 13(4):354–365.

Innes, A. and Manthorpe, J. (2013) Developing theoretical understandings of dementia and their application to dementia care policy in the United Kingdom (UK). *Dementia* 12(6):682–696.

Innes, A., Morgan, D. and Kostenieuk, J. (2011) Informal dementia care in rural and remote settings: A systematic review. *Maturitas* 68(1):34–46.

Jacques, A. and Jackson, G. (2000) *Understanding Dementia*. Edinburgh: Churchill Livingstone.

Koch, T. and Iliffe, S. (2010) Rapid appraisal of barriers to the diagnosis and management of patients with dementia in primary care: A systematic review. *BMC Family Practice* 11:52.

La Fontaine, J., Ahuja J., Bradbury N., Phillips S. and Oyebode J. (2007) Understanding dementia amongst people in minority ethnic and cultural groups. *Journal of Advanced Nursing* 60:605–614.

Laron, M., Mannheim, I., Brodsky, J., Sternberg, S., Zalomonson, S., PlaeucuKertesz, D. and Shefet, D. (2018) Barriers and enablers to timely diagnosis of dementia: Patients' and families' points of view. *Alzheimer's and Dementia* 14(7):P1642. https://doi.org/10.1016/j.jalz.2018.06.3002

Manthrope, J., Iliffe, S. and Eden, A. (2003) Early recognition of dementia by nurses. *Journal of Advanced Nursing* 42(2):183–191.

Manthorpe, J., Samsi, K., Campbell, S., Abley, C., Keady, J., Bond, J. and Iliffe, S. (2013) From forgetfulness to dementia: Clinical and commissioning implications of diagnostic experiences. *British Journal of General Practice* 63(606):e69–e75.

Maslow, K., Selstaad, J. and Denman, S. (2002) Guidelines and care management issues for people with Alzheimer's disease and other dementias. *Disease Management and Health Outcomes* 10(11):693–706.

McCleary, L., Persaud, M., Hum, S., Pimlott, N.J.G., Cohen, C.A., Koehn, S., Leung, K.K., Dalziel, W.B., Kozak, J., Emerson, V.F., Silvius, J.L., Garcia, L. and Drummond, N. (2012) Pathways to dementia diagnosis among South Asian Canadians. *Dementia: The International Journal of Social Research and Practice* 12:769–789. doi: 10.1177/1471301212444806

Milne, A.J. (2000) Early diagnosis of dementia by GPs: An exploratory study of attitudes. *Aging and Mental Health* 4(4):292–300.

Milne, A.J., Woolford, H.H., Mason, J. and Hatzidimitriadou, E. (2000) Early diagnosis of dementia by GPs: An exploratory study of attitudes. *Aging & Mental Health* 4(4):292–300. doi: 10.1080/713649958

Morgan, T. and Crowder, R. (2003) Mini mental state examinations in English: Are they suitable for people with dementia who are Welsh speaking? *Dementia* 2(2):267–272(6).

National Audit Office (2007) Improving services and support for people with dementia. https://www.nao.org.uk/wp-content/uploads/2007/07/0607604.pdf

Parker, M., Barlow, S., Hoe, J. and Aitken, L. (2020). Persistent barriers and facilitators to seeking help for a dementia diagnosis: A systematic review of 30 years of the perspectives of carers and people with dementia. *International Psychogeriatrics* 1–24. doi: 10.1017/S1041610219002229

Phillips, J., Pond, C.D., Paterson, N.E., Howell, C., Shell, A., Stocks, N.P., Goode, S.M. and Marley, J.E. (2012) Difficulties in disclosing the diagnosis of dementia: A qualitative study in general practice. *British Journal of General Practice* 62(601):e546-e553. doi: 10.3399/bjgp12X653598

Pratt, R., Clare, L. and Kirchner, V. (2006) "It's like a revolving door syndrome": Professional perspectives on models of access to services for people with early-stage dementia. *Aging and Mental Health* 10(1):55–62.

Pratt, R. and Wilkinson, H. (2003) A psychosocial model of understanding the experience of receiving a diagnosis of dementia. *Dementia* 2(2):181–199.

Rait, G. (2000) Validating screening instruments for cognitive impairment in older South Asians in the United Kingdom. *International Journal of Geriatric Psychiatry* 15:54–62.

Rimmer, A. (2016) BMA meeting: Early dementia diagnosis is pointless without support services. *BMJ: British Medical Journal* 353. doi: 10.1136/bmj.i3505

Robinson, L., Bamford, C., Briel, R., Spencer, J. and Whitty, P. (2010) Improving patient-centered care for people with dementia in medical encounters: An educational intervention for old age psychiatrists. *International Psychogeriatrics* 22(1):129–138.

Robinson, L., Tang, E. and Taylor, J.P. (2015) Dementia: Timely diagnosis and early intervention (Clinical Review). *BMJ* 350. https://doi.org/10.1136/bmj.h3029

Sagbakken, M., Spilker, R.S. and Nielsen, T.R. (2018) Dementia and immigrant groups: A qualitative study of challenges related to identifying, assessing, and diagnosing dementia. *BMC Health Services Research* 18:910. https://doi.org/10.1186/s12913-018-3720-7

Scottish Government (2008) HEAT Target 4. Improvement in the early diagnosis and management of patients with dementia. http://www.scotland.gov.uk/Topics/Health/health/mentalhealth/servicespolicy/DFMH/antidepressantprescribing

Speechly, C.M., Bridges-Webb, C. and Passmore, E. (2009) The pathway to dementia diagnosis. *Medical Journal of Australia* 189(9): 487–489.

Turner, S., Iliffe, S., Downs, M., Bryans, M., Wilcock, J. and Austin, T. (2003) Decision support software for dementia diagnosis and management in primary care: Relevance and potential. *Aging & Mental Health* 7(1):28–33. doi: 10.1080/1360789021000058148

van den Dungen, P., van Kuijk, L., van Marwijk, H., van der Wouden, J., van Charante, E.M., van der Horst, H. and van Hout, H. (2014)

Preferences regarding disclosure of a diagnosis of dementia: A systematic review. *International Psychogeriatrics* 26(10):1603–1618.

Walker, I.F., Lord, P.A. and Farragher, T.M (2017) Variations in dementia diagnosis in England and association with general practice characteristics. *Primary Health Care Research and Development* 18(3):235–241. doi: 10.1017/S146342361700007X

Watson, R., Bryant, J., Sanson-Fisher, R., Mansfield, E. and Evans, T.J. (2018) What is a "timely" diagnosis? Exploring the preferences of Australian health service consumers regarding when a diagnosis of dementia should be disclosed. *BMC Health Services Research*. https://doi.org/10.1186/s12913-018-3409-y

Werner, P., Karnieli-Miller, O. and Eidelman, S. (2013) Current knowledge and future directions about the disclosure of dementia: A systematic review of the first decade of the 21st century. *Alzheimers Dementia* 9(2):e74–e88.

Woods, B., Arosio, F., Diaz, A., Gove, D., Holmerová, I., Kinnaird, L., Mátlová, M., Okkonen, E., Possenti, M., Roberts, J., Salmi, A., Buuse, S., Werkman, W. and Georges, J. (2019) Timely diagnosis of dementia? Family carers' experiences in 5 European countries. *International Journal of Geriatric Psychiatry* 34(1):114–121.

World Health Organisation (2012) *Dementia a Public Health Priority*. Geneva: World Health Orgnisation.

Xanthopoulou, P., Dooley, J., Meo, I. and Bass, N. (2019) Patient and companion concerns when receiving a dementia diagnosis: An observational study of dementia diagnosis feedback meetings. *Ageing and Society*. https://doi.org/10.1017/s0144686x18000247

Zaleta, A.K. and Carpenter, B.D. (2010) Patient-centered communication during the disclosure of a dementia diagnosis. *American Journal of Alzheimer's Disease and Other Dementias* 25(6):513–520.

SECTION 2
POST-DIAGNOSTIC SUPPORT

After receiving the diagnosis of dementia, individuals may need time to process the information, work out what this might mean for them and start to explore the types of services and supports that may be available to them. This can be a period of great change for individuals as they adjust to what living with dementia might mean for them. It also is a time when relatives, friends and partners of the person with dementia may need assistance as they adjust to their role and acquire the skills and knowledge they need to take on support roles that they had not expected and are not necessarily prepared for.

Post-diagnostic support is an area that has deservedly received much attention and there is a lot of information available, with many studies designed to explore the impact or benefits to people living with dementia and/or their care supporters. This section has three chapters. Chapter 3 will first examine the post-diagnostic support needs of people living with dementia. Chapter 4 will then examine the post-diagnostic support needs for family members and other care supporters. In chapter 5 we will consider initiatives designed to support both the person living with dementia and their care partners together.

3

POST-DIAGNOSTIC SUPPORT FOR THE PERSON LIVING WITH DEMENTIA

Research demonstrates that keeping physically, socially and mentally active are all important when it comes to living well with dementia. However, what this might mean in practice will vary as each individual diagnosed with dementia will have their own interests (politics, religious observances, creative pursuits, cultural pursuits), hobbies (knitting, woodwork, sports, model building, flower arranging) and preferences in how they spend their recreational time (mental stimulation, social stimulation and physical stimulation).

Person-centred (Kitwood, 1997; Brooker and Letham, 2016) or individualised care approaches (Mendes, 2015) have the individual firmly at the centre of developing support packages designed to promote the wellbeing of each individual. However, putting such approaches into practice can be challenging, with limited resources available. Within whatever fiscal or practical challenges one may face, it is important to remember that each person is unique and will have their own characteristics, history and preferences. They will also have their own routines (for example when they get up, a daily walk, meeting friends and family) and responsibilities (feeding the fish, cutting the grass, cleaning the home, visiting friends, child care). It is important that each individual is supported in maintaining their sense of self via opportunities to remain socially, mentally and physically active, but also has the chance to learn new things, join new groups and generally remain an active participant in social life.

A social citizenship model (Hughes, 2019; Brannelly, 2016; Bartlett and O'Connor, 2007) has been growing in popularity in the dementia field. There is an articulated desire from policy makers (Department of Health, 2012), practitioners and of course, people living with dementia themselves who campaign for change and inclusion (Bowker et al., 2020; Bartlett, 2014), that is, for those with dementia to be recognised as active social participants who have rights and are able to participate actively in their communities. There is a clearly articulated view amongst people living with dementia that when they are provided with appropriate support or 'scaffolding' (McCabe et al., 2018) to enable their participation in their communities, this can be their reality for as long as possible. One man living with dementia recently eloquently said, 'I do not require a carer, I require a personal assistant to help me live well and independently. My wife is my wife. Not my carer' (personal communication). There are four areas that we will focus on in this chapter:

1   Getting out and about independently.
2   Opportunities to engage with other people living with dementia.
3   Keeping physically active.
4   Advance care planning.

We will conclude this section with the story, in her own words, of the post-diagnostic support experience of a person living with dementia, Lesley Calvert.

GETTING OUT AND ABOUT INDEPENDENTLY

A combination of factors may unfortunately begin to limit the ability of people living with dementia to continue to get out and about on their own. These could be due to other health conditions and physical mobility restrictions, or due to cognitive decline, or a lack of transport options that if not addressed creatively could lead to social isolation.

Driving

A decision is often made to remove the driving license of the person diagnosed with dementia, and this can be devastating both in terms of a feeling of loss of ability, and also the loss of the means to remain independent in the way that they have until their diagnosis. In a comprehensive study of professionals' attitudes towards fitness to drive (Hawley, 2010), it was found that there were gaps in knowledge and processes, and confusion as to whose responsibility it is to raise the topic of fitness to drive. To address this confusion guidelines on driving and dementia have been developed and now exist for clinicians to consult when beginning to consider if an individual with dementia may need to review their driving (e.g. Taylor et al., 2018). The process of developing such guidelines, for example the Canadian National Guidelines on Driving and Dementia, has been one that has been developed sensitively and thoroughly through careful consideration of the complexities of this issue (Rapaport et al., 2018). However, although the processes exist to help determine whether a person with dementia is safe to drive, the feelings experienced by an individual with dementia arising from no longer being able to drive can be profound.

James McKillop (2016) provides a personal account of his experience about how he had to stop driving and how the desire to drive has never left him. He provides a really innovative example of how he was enabled to drive again during a supervised session on an airfield! He talks about a variety of ways he may try in the future to once again feel the power of an engine at his fingertips. However, his account provides a clear expression of his frustration, resentment and sense of loss that occurred when his driving license was not renewed. His experience indicates the sensitivity that those communicating this decision need to have when discussing and withdrawing what may be the primary means of feeling independent an individual may have.

Public transport

Public transport may appear to be the solution to not being able to drive, but this will depend on the quality and quantity of the services available where someone lives. Those in cities may find it easier to adjust to not being able to drive if they can access other means of transportation. However, those living in remote or rural areas may find that their options to get around radically impact upon their ability to access everyday services such as hospitals, shops and banks if they can no longer drive. In Scotland, an initiative known as

'Upstream' (Hyde and Cassidy, 2017) has explored the barriers and solutions to enabling people living with dementia to travel. Barriers include:

1 People losing their confidence.
2 Becoming anxious or feeling unsafe.
3 The complexities involved in independent travel can be confusing (from reading a timetable, to finding the correct payment, to finding the correct bus stop or train platform).
4 Inequalities resulting from difficulties paying online or accessing special rates and fares.
5 Lack of knowledge about potential support available.

Based on work with people living with dementia in different Scottish regions, potential solutions to travelling with dementia were identified as:

1 Providing training to those who may be able to offer support to people living with dementia who are travelling.
2 Developing community transport initiatives.
3 Providing staff with a visual prompt that the person in front of them may need special assistance (e.g. via a lanyard system often used in airports for those who have requested assistance to travel).
4 Ensuring service providers are aware of the issues that people living with dementia have shared as barriers to travelling.

In a guide produced by the Scottish Dementia Group Working Transport Group, comprised of members of the Scottish Dementia Working Group (2013), Nancy MacAdam and her colleagues provide an overview of the various modes of transport that people living with dementia may use, such as car, taxi, bus, underground, ferry or plane, and provide suggested tips about how to navigate these different forms of transport. This is an excellent resource for people living with dementia, written by people living with dementia.

Taxis and community transport schemes may be available in some areas with special arrangements for people who have been assessed as needing support to maintain their physical mobility and independence. However, problems using public transport exist, as Lesley's recent experience of using taxis in the Manchester area demonstrates.

Lesley's experience of taxis

When you have dementia it's hard to travel alone, so travelling by taxi is essential.

However, this can be very stressful when the taxi driver doesn't drop you at the place you are going. I was in a taxi to Manchester University. The taxi driver stopped in a bus lane and said 'Get out – you are here'. I said 'but we haven't drove through the barrier'. That was the only thing I remember the person who had booked my taxi mentioning. He got really angry telling me to get out. I was very tearful. Luckily for me, my husband, who couldn't come with me because he was terminally ill, had put the tutor's telephone number in my top pocket. I handed my phone to the taxi driver and said ring this number, which he did and then took me to where I should have been dropped off. I cried for hours and couldn't talk about what I had been asked to talk about. Another time I went with another person who also has dementia to Manchester and when we got there the taxi driver asked us for £20, we both said the taxi had been prebooked and paid for but he insisted we had to pay, so we did. He also put us out of the taxi away from where we were going. Once again I was panicking as we didn't know the area. When we finally got to where we were supposed to go, we told the person from the Alzheimer's Society they had charged us and they got on to the taxi company. They then refunded the money. Talking to another person with dementia at the conference, we discovered they had also been charged twice. Nobody realises how hard it is to travel alone when you are living with dementia; this is why taxi drivers should be encouraged to be a dementia friend.

Walking

Individuals who may no longer be able to drive, who cannot access public transport for whatever reason or who may be looking for simple solutions that do not require navigating public transport may decide to begin to walk (or cycle) to local amenities such as the corner shop, the post office or their local health centre. However, over time their ability to way-find may decline, resulting in both the person with dementia and their families being concerned as to where it is safe for the person to travel to unaccompanied, whether it is on foot or using public transport. Safe zones, that is, areas from which the person with dementia may be able to find their way home unaccompanied, often shrink as dementia progresses, leading to increased feelings of frustration and isolation. Being unable to get out and about independently will also impact on the person with dementia relying on others for assistance and support with what was a taken for granted aspect of daily life prior to the diagnosis and development of dementia symptoms. Various solutions may be found, for example, tracking devices (McCabe and Innes, 2013) can offer the person with dementia peace of mind that if they do go out unaccompanied they have a device that can be used by their families and friends to locate them. For example, GPS tracking on mobile phones may already allow for this, or specially purchased devices with panic alarms that the person with dementia can press if they become lost. Or, if families and friends are already attending an event or going to a place that the person wishes to attend, they may be able to walk or travel together as a solution.

Retaining a sense of independence, even if in a more limited way than before dementia, is an important issue to consider for people living with dementia and their families. Creative thinking may be required to facilitate this, but is likely to enable the person to live at home for longer. Additionally, families and care supporters may be able to continue with their support roles for longer if they can have respite from constant care responsibilities and also peace of mind that the person with dementia is safe.

OPPORTUNITIES TO ENGAGE AND INTERACT WITH OTHER PEOPLE LIVING WITH DEMENTIA

One of the most commonly reported positives of attending groups designed for people living with dementia is the opportunity to be with others who understand their situation and who they can share experiences and tips for coping with and adjusting to changes in abilities and everyday functioning (Bowker et al., 2020). This may come about through attending different kinds of groups and activities that are for people with similar conditions and circumstances, or from people living with dementia joining forces as activists and agitators for change. We will consider both forms of engagement in turn.

Psychosocial groups and interventions for people living with dementia

There is now a massive amount of literature (McDermott et al., 2019) that looks at different forms of *psychosocial approaches* (Moniz-Cook et al., 2011) to promoting wellbeing for people living with dementia. Psychosocial approaches are in essence those that seek to provide social and mental stimulation and support to the person living with dementia and/or their care supporters. They have often been seen as a way to bring about benefit to the lives of people with dementia in the absence of a cure via drug therapies. In a useful commentary on psychosocial approaches, Oyebode and Parveen (2019) found that the appointment of dementia specialists and attention to case management can produce positive outcomes; physical therapies, cognitive training and modified cognitive behaviour therapy also had a range of benefits. They found that interventions tended to be short term with impact only measured in the short term, reflecting the time-limited funding for the initiatives and the short-term nature of the evaluations exploring the impact or benefits for participants. However, a common problem with the research on psychosocial interventions is perceived to be the research design that does not follow the same approach as would commonly be used to evaluate the effectiveness of a drug treatment (Moniz-Cook et al., 2011; Oyebode and Parveen, 2019). This makes it difficult for the value of small scale, short term or local initiatives to be seen as having benefit to people living with dementia.

Yet talking to people living with dementia and reading empirical studies exploring the views and experiences of people living with dementia tells us that those living with the diagnosis perceive the opportunity to engage and interact with others as hugely beneficial. Individuals with dementia participating in schemes designed to provide one-on-one support to enable them to access activities of their choice report enjoying the benefits such support brings (Kelly and Innes, 2014). Gaining access to support post-diagnosis can reduce the risk of social isolation and exclusion for people living in remote and rural areas (Innes et al., 2014) and there are many practice-based examples, with practitioners sharing the benefits of different types of groups for people living with dementia in journals such as *The Journal of Dementia Care* and the Practice section in *Dementia*. All ably demonstrate the power and impact of finding ways to engage, include and encourage participation in groups and topics as varied as the ways each of us might choose to spend our recreational or leisure time.

Those facilitating group activities report seeing the benefits for people 'in the moment' during their participation in groups that are designed with the intention of social inclusion and promoting well-being (Scholar et al., 2019). These in-the-moment experiences may be as or more important than a prolonged benefit that a traditional research design of a clinical trial seeks to capture. A person living with dementia may over time not remember the 'in the moment' experiences but enjoyment, relaxation and stimulation may result in better sleep, less anxiety and agitation and an overall increase in enjoyment of life. Such approaches are crucial lifelines for people living with dementia to remain connected to their communities and to remain active in areas that interest them.

There is a plethora of examples of the types of groups available to people living with dementia. Those that that have been reported positively by people living with dementia include:

1   Cafés stemming from the Alzheimer Café movement in the Netherlands designed to offer peer support and information-sharing opportunities.
2   Outdoor activities, such as gardening, walking or sports.
3   Interest-specific groups, for example crafts or technology.
4   Activities involving music.
5   Initiatives designed to promote social inclusion via the arts, including museums, galleries and heritage sites.
6   Activities designed to promote physical activity.

There have also been initiatives to target specific groups who may not always be enthusiastic about attending traditional types of services or groups. For example groups targeting men with dementia (Hicks et al., 2019) were found to be successful as reported by the participants because they were able to spend time with other men from their local communities. There have also been efforts to create groups in the areas where people live, so that people don't have to travel to an urban centre. In farming groups in rural areas (Bruin et al., 2017; Ibsen et al., 2018) and community gardening groups (Noone et al., 2015; Noone and Jenkins, 2018), participants have reported a sense of belonging and participation.

Coming together to agitate for change

There are individuals who want to come together not just to socialise, have fun, interact and enjoy an activity or group. Rather, they wish to bring about change and improvements in their lives and others' lives who may be affected by dementia in the future. In recognition of the part people living with dementia have to play in influencing thinking about dementia, Alzheimer Disease International (2012) developed guidelines for supporting people with dementia to speak publicly about their experiences.

Many working groups now exist at regional, national and international levels and serve as examples of work by dedicated and determined individuals who inspire others to consider their experiences and what this means for those developing policy, practice and research. The work of the Scottish Dementia Working Group is particularly well established and has helped to shape Scottish policy around dementia (Weaks et al., 2012). There are numerous examples now of how people living with dementia are core to the research agenda (Swarbrick et al., 2016).

Activist and advocacy groups for people living with dementia

Regional

> Open Doors www.dementiavoices.org.uk/group/open-doors-project/

National

> DEEP www.dementiavoices.org.uk/about-deep/
>
> Scottish Dementia Working Group www.alzscot.org/our-work/campaigning-for-change/have-your-say/scottish-dementia-working-group
>
> 3 Nations Dementia Working Group www.alzheimers.org.uk/get-involved/engagement-participation/three-nations-dementia-working-group
>
> Irish Dementia Working Group https://alzheimer.ie/creating-change/self-advocacy-groups/irish-dementia-working-group/

International

European Working Group of People with Dementia www.alzheimer-europe.org/Alzheimer-Europe/Who-we-are/European-Working-Group-of-People-with-Dementia

Dementia Advocacy and Support Network International www.dasninternational.org/

Research has demonstrated that people with dementia can find a sense of power in a collective identity when they first come to terms with, adapt and adjust to what living with dementia means for them (Clare et al., 2008), and this may be particularly well achieved via a common 'cause' or agenda to promote change (Rochford-Brennan, 2020). People with dementia actively manage their presentation of self to the external world (Birt et al., 2019) to ensure they can continue to maintain their social connections and relations with the wider social world. Ruth Bartlett (2014) asked 16 people living with dementia about their campaigning work, and although this was valued, it was demanding and took its toll on individuals physically and mentally. It takes effort, stamina and determination to cope with a condition and drive a change agenda forward.

Bringing about change can also be achieved via raising awareness of what it means to live with dementia. Public performances showcasing skills have been found to be a powerful way to challenge negative perceptions of what it means to live with dementia (Reynolds et al., 2016), but public-facing work can be an exhausting experience (Bartlett, 2014). The impact of hearing a person with dementia speak about the policy, practice or research issues that need to be addressed to ensure their needs are at the fore is perhaps one of the most powerful ways to bring about change. People often express surprise that the person with dementia can function so well, and therefore demonstrate a lack of insight into the toll it takes for a person with dementia to speak up publicly. However, it has become the norm at international meetings such as those organised by Alzheimer Europe and Alzheimer Disease International for people living with dementia to have sessions where they share what is happening in their part of the world and learn from one another about how they might bring about change that is meaningful to them.

KEEPING PHYSICALLY ACTIVE

Evidence on the importance of physical activity for prevention and delay of long-term conditions is strong. Activity rates are known to decline substantially particularly around later life, yet remaining physically active can have cognitive benefits (Olanrewaju et al., 2016). The research evidence consistently demonstrates the benefits of keeping physically active to maintain abilities once dementia has been diagnosed (Hulme et al., 2010), and the evidence suggests that physical activity for people living with dementia has benefits not only in reducing agitation and lethargy, but also improving fitness, function and mood (Bowes et al., 2013). Learning how to maintain or increase levels of physical activity and exercise as part of a post-diagnostic support plan is important, yet there are many identified barriers to achieving this in practice (van Alphen et al., 2016). These have been grouped as:

- *Interpersonal* – dependence on others to facilitate.
- *Intrapersonal* – other health and mobility issues an individual may have that need to be overcome.
- *Community* – barriers included working out the transportation to where exercise activities may be available, a lack of dedicated space, bad weather and lack of specifically designed exercise programs.

(Van Alphen et al., 2016)

In Canadian research, the approach and support of family members to motivate the person with dementia to be physically active (Dal Bello Haas et al., 2014) can be crucial in maintaining or improving levels of physical activity. In Australia, Cations et al. (2019) found that clinicians have difficulty delivering exercise-based interventions to overcome the identified barriers. This means that despite policy drivers and best practice guidelines that support exercise and physical activity interventions for people living with dementia, it can be difficult to access formal support in this way.

People can therefore be encouraged to be creative in their approach to remaining physically active. The benefits to general physical health may help maintain an individual's ability to remain independent for longer. Physical activity can also be part of a social outing, for example, dog and other walking groups, attending sports events such as golf, cricket or football team events and yoga and other mind-body activities that may also promote mental wellbeing as well as the physical benefits of taking part in an exercise group. Exercising outside has been shown to have benefits (Gladwell et al., 2013), with connections to nature having further therapeutic benefits; things like gardening or working in an allotment may all have even more benefits than simply keeping physically active.

Guides aimed at people living with dementia about how to keep physically active and generally keep healthy provide useful ideas about the types of activities that may have general health benefits and that may benefit people living with dementia (Age Scotland, 2018). However, these activities may be limited by the ability to get out and about independently and the availability of services and groups where an individual lives.

PLANNING FOR THE FUTURE

People living with dementia may want assistance in thinking about their support and care preferences as their symptoms and needs develop over time. We will discuss changing and increasing needs in chapter 6 and end of life care support in chapter 7, but it is important to acknowledge that post-diagnostic support also entails looking to the future as well as maintaining levels of wellbeing and abilities.

Advance care planning offers a way for people to document the wishes of the person living with dementia while they are still able to articulate and contribute to discussions, and therefore retain some control over what may happen to them if their care needs grow over time. In their review of literature relating to advanced care planning, Dening et al. (2011) identified that there are low numbers of formal advance care plans for people living with dementia and that the time available to develop these is often limited due to changes in cognition that can occur. They argued that this is an area requiring further education for all involved as it is likely that, as with other conditions and diagnoses, the more knowledge and education professionals and families have, the more likely they will be able to support the person living with dementia to think ahead and plan for the future. When looking at advance care planning for people living with dementia in care homes, Robinson et al., (2012) concluded that it was too late to conduct such work in care homes because the majority of people were deemed to be lacking in capacity by this point. Therefore, there was very little impact on outcomes for people living with dementia as it was too late to adequately gain and document their views and preferences. Time is of the essence, yet planning for future declines in ability or increase in support needs is not necessarily what those who have recently been diagnosed may wish to think about as they initially navigate the system and seek out information and early support to continue to live as well as possible.

There is a limited body of work that looks at advance care planning from the perspective of people living with dementia. One such exception is work by Dickinson et al. (2013) where they examined people living with dementia and their families' views on care planning. They found that there were a number of barriers to individuals completing formal advance care plans:

1   Lack of knowledge and awareness.
2   Difficulty in finding the right time to discuss and work out what their preferences may be.
3   A preference for informal plans discussed with families rather than written documentation.
4   Lack of perceived choices around future care.
5   Lack of support to make choices about future health care.

Dickinson et al. (2013) found that financial planning was most likely to formalised, but that other areas of care and support needs tended to be discussed informally, if at all.

The general practitioner is often the health professional that a person with dementia has the most contact with; therefore, they may be well placed to begin discussions about future planning. In a systematic review, Tilburgs et al. (2018) demonstrated that the earlier general practitioners can facilitate the discussion with the person with dementia about their future care and support preferences the better, as delays in doing this may result in some individuals being unable to be consulted about their wishes while they still have the ability to be involved in future planning. People with dementia are likely to be more receptive to considering future care needs when they are aware it is about ensuring they have as normal a life as possible that takes account of their preferences and views. Looking at the role of primary care more generally and the role those working in memory clinics may have in supporting the development of advance care plans with people living with dementia in the community, Lee et al. (2019) found that staff rated the importance of advance care plans highly but had more limited knowledge and that only around 40 percent of those attending these primary care memory clinics had an advance care plan. This disconnect adds to the growing calls for more education for everyone who could contribute to taking this area of post-diagnostic support forward.

Post-diagnostic support for people living with dementia will naturally focus on the immediate needs of people living with dementia, but it is important to use this time to also consider the future and to plan where possible in a way that ensures the views and preferences of the individual living with dementia will continue to be heard. We will return to these issues in chapters 6 and 7.

Lesley's story

After I was diagnosed, and I had been finished from work, we needed to know what services were available. This was in November. Luckily there was a small 'pop-up' van on Salford precinct from the Alzheimer's Society, so my husband and I went in and the young lady said she would come to our house and let us know what was available in our area. She steered us towards the Humphrey Booth Resource Centre in Swinton.

Humphrey Booth told us that in the new year there would be a post-diagnostic support group run by Greater Manchester West Mental Health Team, and if we were interested we could put our name down and the team would get in touch when the course was starting. At the end of January we were contacted and two of the people running the course came to the house and explained about the course.

This course was just what we needed. It was once a week for six weeks and we met other couples in the same position. The course explained the difference between dementia and Alzheimer's, also it explained about power of attorney, medications and other groups that were running in the city for people living with dementia and their carers. They also said that it was essential to keep active and eat a healthy diet, as this helped the brain. One of the sessions we were at split the people living with dementia in one group and the carers in the other. I felt this was a really good session as it enabled us both to talk freely about what was worrying us without it upsetting each other.

There was a lot to take in, but we made some great friends. These people are still our friends and we meet them once a month at Open Doors, run by Greater Manchester Mental Health at the Humphrey Booth Resource Centre. You are entitled to come to this group after the six-week course.

At one of the meetings at Humphrey Booth I was asked if I was interested in a piece of research about keeping fit and healthy for people living with dementia, as I wasn't getting much exercise, and because I wasn't working I decided to take them up on the offer. I really enjoyed this piece of research and I met more people from around Manchester who had dementia. They say that if you stay fit and healthy it helps the dementia, so that has been my aim from the start.

From that first meeting after the six-week course I found out about other groups. We joined the Dementia Champions group run by the CCG (Clinical Commissioning Group). This group set up the Steps document in Salford, which takes you through the journey from going to your GP to what to do after a diagnosis of dementia. We meet once a month and have been asked to help with many more projects about dementia.

One of the first groups I was involved with was a group for people who were diagnosed with dementia under the age of 65. There were about six people with dementia and their carers. We first met at Eccles Gateway with a couple of people from Age UK Salford to set up this new group. It is still running today at Mount Chapel Church Hall and is called MCC (Mount Chapel Champions) and now has over 40 members.

One of the best projects was when they asked us about setting up a Dementia Swim. I told them it was no use asking me, as I had a fear of water so couldn't swim. I was told they would teach me to swim. So, as I am game for anything, I went along. They wanted the swim to be dementia friendly so it was suggested we had a pool attendant just for the people with dementia to keep them safe. We also wanted it to be a place to meet different people so after the swim we would have a drink and something to eat in the café. This was an achievement for me as I went from a non-swimmer to being able to swim 64 lengths in just over an hour. Although the Dementia Swim has now finished I still go to the swimming pool at least once a week, but sometimes more. It is something I would never had thought of doing without being diagnosed with dementia.

Next, I joined the Associates at Salford University. We helped with the planning of the new Dementia Hub, from the colour scheme to the chairs and tables and the signage. It was a great achievement as we had been asked from the beginning to help. The hub was opened in May 2017 by Christopher Eccleston. Associates help students who need to know about dementia as part of their course. One student was studying photography and she took photographs of me swimming. This photograph is on the wall in the Dementia Hub, with other photographs she took of people living with dementia and carers doing the thing they enjoyed. We have also spoken at nursing conferences and other university conferences.

On the first Monday of the month is SIDS Café at the University of Salford. We needed a name for the café instead of just calling it a dementia café, as dementia still has a stigma. My husband Sam thought of SIDS Café, which stands for Salford Institute for Dementia. The people living with dementia or the carers suggest activities so that we don't get bored doing the same thing. We have made bouquets of chocolates, painted stones which people take and put in the local parks and many other different activities.

I thought when I was diagnosed with Alzheimer's my life was over – but I now have a new lease on life. I sometimes wonder how I had time to work!

I find something to do most days which keeps me connected. I think my dementia would have deteriorated more quickly if I didn't get to associate with different people in different places as I would have been isolated in my home, especially after the death of my husband. Social stimulation is important, and perhaps social prescribing should be used more than prescriptions for medication, such as when people who get depressed and are given antidepressants.

It is a shame that a number of groups that were set up have closed because of lack of funding. People living with dementia like routine, so to set up a club and then a few months later stop it really doesn't help us. In my view, there is nothing better than going out, socialising and talking to people.

Hearing the voices of people living with dementia is important as it provides insights into what it may be like in the future for those recently diagnosed and also for those providing care and support.

Web resource illustrating living with dementia

This weblink takes you to a short video intended to illustrate what it may be like to live with dementia:

www.scie.org.uk/dementia/about/dementia-from-the-inside.asp

There are many guides now available to assist people as they adjust to their diagnosis and continue to live their lives with dementia. Accessing these is a good first step. Direct support from others living with dementia and those who provide or facilitate support and services/initiatives is another way to learn more about dementia and to also have fun along the way.

Online sources of information and support

Online resources abound with tips and ideas about living well with dementia after receiving the diagnosis, here are a few that we think are a good starting point:

Alzheimer Society www.alzheimers.org.uk/get-support/daily-living/ staying-healthy-dementia
Canadian Alzheimer Association https://alzheimer.ca/en/Home/ About-dementia/Brain-health/Be-socially-active
Northern Ireland Direct Government Services www.nidirect.gov. uk/articles/staying-mentally-active
Social Care Institute for Excellence www.scie.org.uk/dementia/ living-with-dementia/keeping-active/

REFERENCES

Age Scotland (2018) *Healthy Living and Dementia*. www.ageuk.org. uk/globalassets/age-scotland/documents/ia---factsheets/dementia/ dem-4-dementia-and-healthy-living-jan-2018.pdf

Alzheimer's Disease International (2012) *How to Successfully Involve People with Dementia in Speaking Roles for Organisations*. London: Alzheimer's Disease International.

Bartlett, R. (2014) Citizenship in action: The lived experiences of citizens with dementia who campaign for social change. *Disability and Society* 29(8):1291–1304. https://doi.org/10.1080/09687599.2014.924905

Bartlett, R. and O'Connor, D. (2007) From personhood to citizenship: Broadening the lens for dementia practice and research. *Journal of Aging Studies* 21(2):107–118. https://doi.org/10.1016/j.jaging.2006.09.002

Birt, L., Griffiths, R., Charlesworth, G., Higgs, P., Orrell, M., Leung, P. and Poland, F. (2019) Maintaining social connections in dementia: A qualitative synthesis. *Qualitative Health Research*. doi: 10.1177/1049732319874782

Bowes, A., Dawson, A., Jepson, R. and McCabe, L. (2013) Physical activity for people with dementia: A scoping study. *BMC Geriatrics* 13. doi: 10.1186/1471-2318-13-129

Bowker, R., Calvert, L., Allcroft, F., Bowker, G., Foy, P., Gandy, J., Jones, S., Bushell, S., Clark, A. and Innes, A. (2020) "Our voice started off as a whisper and now it is a great big roar": The Salford Dementia Associate Panel as a model of involvement in research activities. *Dementia* 19(1):18–26. doi: 10.1177/1471301219874225

Brannelly, T. (2016) Citizenship and people living with dementia: A case for the ethics of care. *Dementia*. https://doi.org/10.1177/1471301216639463

Brooker, D. and Letham, I. (2016) *Person Centred Care: Making Services Better with the VIP Framework* (2nd edition). London: Jessica Kingsley.

Bruin, S.D., Boer, B.D., Beerens, H., Buist, Y. and Verbeek, H. (2017) Rethinking dementia care: The value of green care farming. *The Journal of Post-Acute and Long-Term Care Medicine* 18(3):200–203. https://doi.org/10.1016/j.jamda.2016.11.018

Cations, M., Radisic, G., de la Perrelle, L. and Laver, K.E. (2019) Post-diagnostic allied health interventions for people with dementia in Australia: A spotlight on current practice. *BMC Research Notes* 12. doi: 10.1186/s13104-019-4588-2

Clare, L., Rowlands, J. and Quin, R. (2008) Collective strength: The impact of developing a shared social identity in early-stage dementia. *Dementia: The International Journal of Social Research and Practice* 7:9–30. doi: 10.1177/1471301207085365

Dal Bello-Haas, V.P.M., O'Connell, M.E., Morgan, D.G. and Cross-ley, M. (2014) Lessons learned: Feasibility and acceptability of a telehealth-delivered exercise intervention for rural-dwelling individuals with dementia and their caregivers. *Rural and Remote Health* 14:2715.

Dening, K., Jones, L. and Sampson, E. (2011) Advance care planning for people with dementia: A review. *International Psychogeriatrics* 23(10):1535–1551.

Department of Health (2012) *Prime Minister's Challenge on Dementia*. London. https://assets.publishing.service.gov.uk/government/uploads/system/uploads/attachment_data/file/215101/dh_133176.pdf

Dickinson, C., Bamford, C., Exley, C., Emmett, C., Hughes, J. and Robinson, L. (2013) Planning for tomorrow whilst living for today: The views of people with dementia and their families on advance care planning. *International Psychogeriatrics* 25(12). https://doi.org/10.1017/S1041610213001531

Gladwell, V.F., Brown, D.K., Wood, C., Sandercock, G.R. and Barton, J.L. (2013) The great outdoors: How a green exercise environment can benefit all. *Extreme Physiology & Medicine* 2(1):3.

Hawley, C. (2010) The Attitudes of Health Professionals to Giving Advice on Fitness to Drive. London: Department for Transport. www.dft.gov.uk/pgr/roadsafety/research/rsrr/theme6/report91/

Hicks, B., Innes, A. and Nyman, S.R. (2019) Exploring the "active mechanisms" for engaging rural-dwelling older men with dementia in a community technological initiative. *Ageing and Society*:1–33. doi: 10.1017/S0144686X19000357

Hughes, J.C. (2019) Citizenship and authenticity in dementia: A scoping review. *Maturitas*. doi: 10.1016/j.maturitas.2019.04.001

Hulme, C., Wright, J., Crocker, T., Oluboyede, Y. and House, A. (2010) Non-pharmacological approaches for dementia that informal carers might try or access: A systematic review. *International Journal of Geriatric Psychiatry* 25:756–763. doi: 10.1002/gps.2429

Hyde, A. and Cassidy, S. (2017) *Upstream: Travelling Well with Dementia*. Glasgow: Life Changes Trust. www.lifechangestrust.org.uk/sites/default/files/publications/Upstream%20Final%20Report.pdf

Ibsen, T.L., Eriksen, S. and Patil, G.G. (2018) Farm-based day care in Norway: A complementary service for people with dementia. *Journal Multidisciplinary Healthcare* 11:349–358. doi: 10.2147/JMDH.S167135

Innes, A., Szymczynska, P. and Stark, C. (2014) Dementia diagnosis and post-diagnostic support in Scottish rural communities:

Experiences of people with dementia and their families. *Dementia* 13(2):233–247. doi: 10.1177/1471301212460608

Kelly, F. and Innes, A. (2014) Facilitating independence: The benefits of a post-diagnostic support project for people with dementia. *Dementia*. doi: 10.1177/1471301214520780

Kitwood, T. (1997) *Dementia Reconsidered: The Person Comes First.* Buckingham: Open University Press.

Lee, L., Hillier, L.M., Locklin, J., Lee, J. and Slonim, K. (2019) Advanced care planning for persons with dementia in primary care: Attitudes and barriers among health-care professionals. *Journal of Palliative Care* 34(4):248–254.

McCabe, L and Innes, A. (2013) Supporting safe walking for people with dementia: User participation in the development of new technology. *Gerotechnology* 12(1):4–15. doi:10.4017/gt.2013.12.1.006.00

McCabe, L., Robertson, J. and Kelly, F. (2018) Scaffolding and working together: A qualitative exploration of strategies for everyday life with dementia. *Age and Ageing* 47(2):303–310. doi.org/10.1093/ageing/afx186

McDermott, O., Charlesworth, G., Hogervorst, E., Stoner, C., Moniz-Cook, E., Spector, A., Csipke, E. and Orrell, M. (2019) Psychosocial interventions for people with dementia: A synthesis of systematic reviews. *Aging & Mental Health* 23(4):393–403.

McKillop, J. (2016) *Driving and Dementia: My Experiences.* Glasgow: Life Changes Trust. www.lifechangestrust.org.uk/sites/default/files/Driving%20with%20Dementia%20website.pdf

Mendes, A. (2015) Keeping up with the changing face of individualised dementia care. *Nursing and Residential Care* 17(2). https://doi.org/10.12968/nrec.2015.17.2.100

Moniz-Cook, E., Vernooij-Dassen, M., Woods, B., Orrell, M. and Interdem Network (2011) Psychosocial interventions in dementia care research: The INTERDEM manifesto. *Aging and Mental* 15(3):283–290. https://doi.org/10.1080/13607863.2010.543665

Noone, S., Innes, A., Kelly, F. and Mayers, A. (2015) "The nourishing soil of the soul": The role of horticultural therapy in promoting well-being in community-dwelling people with dementia. *Dementia*. doi: 10.1177/1471301215623889

Noone, S. and Jenkins, N. (2018) Digging for dementia: Exploring the experience of community gardening from the perspectives of people with dementia. *Aging and Mental Health* 22(7):881–888. https://doi.org/10.1080/13607863.2017.139379

Olanrewaju, O., Kelly, S., Cowan, A., Brayne, C. and Lafortune, L. (2016) Physical activity in community-dwelling older people: A review of systematic reviews of interventions and context. (Report) *The Lancet* 388:S83. doi: 10.1016/S0140-6736(16)32319-4

Oyebode, J.R. and Parveen, S. (2019) Psychosocial interventions for people with dementia: An overview and commentary on recent developments. *Dementia* 18(1):8–35.

Rapoport, M.J., Chee, J.N., Carr, D.B., Molnar, F., Naglie, G., Dow, J., Marottoli, R., Mitchell, S., Tant, M., Herrmann, N., Lanctôt, K.L., Taylor, J.P., Donaghy, P.C., Classen, S. and O'Neill, D. (2018) An international approach to enhancing a national guideline on driving and dementia. *Current Psychiatry Repository* 20(3):16. doi: 10.1007/s11920-018–0879-x

Reynolds, L., Innes, A., Poyner, C. and Hambidge, S. (2016) The stigma attached isn't true of real life': Challenging public perception of dementia through a participatory approach involving people with dementia. (Innovative Practice) *Dementia*. doi: 10.1177/147130121663582

Robinson, L., Dickinson, C., Rousseau, N., Beyer, F., Clark, A., Hughes, J., Howel, D. and Exley, C. (2012) A systematic review of the effectiveness of advance care planning interventions for people with cognitive impairment and dementia. *Age and Ageing* 41(2):263–269.

Rochford-Brennan, H. (2020) Living with dementia in rural Ireland. In Innes, A., Morgan, D. and Farmer, J. (Eds.), *Remote and Rural Dementia Care*. Bristol: Policy Press.

Scholar, H., Innes, A., Haragalova, J. and Sharma, S. (2019) "Unlocking the door to being there": The contribution of creative facilitators in supporting people living with dementia to engage with heritage settings. *Dementia*. https://doi.org/10.1177/1471301219871388

Scottish Dementia Working Group's Transport Group (2013) *Travelling with Dementia*. www.lifechangestrust.org.uk/sites/default/files/publications/Travelling-with-dementia-V31.pdf

Swarbrick, C.M., Open Doors, Scottish Dementia Working Group, EDUCATE, Davis, K. and Keady, J. (2016) Visioning change: Co-producing a model of involvement and engagement in research (Innovative Practice). *Dementia*. https://doi.org/10.1177/14713012 16674559

Taylor, J.P., Olsen, K. and Donaghy, P. (2018) *Driving with Dementia or Mild Cognitive Impairment: Consensus Guidelines for Clinicians.* Newcastle: University of Newcastle. https://research.ncl.ac.uk/driving-and-dementia/consensusguidelinesforclinicians/Final%20Guideline.pdf

Tilburgs, B., Vernooij-Dassen, M., Koopmans, R., van Gennip, H., Engels, Y. and Perry, M. (2018) Barriers and facilitators for GPs in dementia advance care planning: A systematic integrative review. *PLoS One* 13(6):e0198535. doi: 10.1371/journal.pone.0198535

van Alphen, H.J.M., Hortobágyi, T. and van Heuvelen, M.J.V. (2016) Barriers, motivators, and facilitators of physical activity in dementia patients: A systematic review. *Archives of Gerontology and Geriatrics* 66:109–118. https://doi.org/10.1016/j.archger.2016.05.008

Weaks, D., Wilkinson, H., Houston, A. and McKillop, J. (2012) *Perspectives on Ageing and Dementia.* York: Joseph Rowntree Foundation.

THE POST-DIAGNOSTIC SUPPORT NEEDS OF FAMILY MEMBERS AND FRIENDS WHO PROVIDE CARE AND SUPPORT

Taking on a support role for the person living with dementia can be a daunting task. It can also become more difficult over time if the person has increased care and support needs that were not initially anticipated. The person providing care may require the support of services and others to enable them to fulfil their care-giving roles.

The person providing care and support will have a range of characteristics that may influence their experiences, for example gender, ethnicity and sexual orientation may all have a bearing on how they experience the support role. The person providing the support may also have health issues and over time can be prone to becoming 'burnt out' if the appropriate supports are not in place to ensure that their needs are also met. There can be both satisfactions and burdens when providing support to a person living with dementia and individual family members and friends will each have their own coping styles and approaches. The experiences of providing support to a person with dementia are not uniform and will vary according to many factors. However, as the person providing support adjusts to their new or newly termed 'carer, caregiver, care partner or care supporter' role, they can experience a number of potential losses (Robinson et al., 2005). We will first consider some of the adjustments and losses.

ADJUSTMENTS AND POTENTIAL LOSSES FOR THOSE PROVIDING CARE AND SUPPORT

It is not just the person living with dementia who has to adjust to their diagnosis, but the people they live with and/or other family members and friends with whom they have close relationships (Robinson et al., 2005). The range of things that an individual care supporter may undertake in their care and support role can vary hugely and can change over time. Supporting someone with dementia may at first only require the care supporter to help with everyday tasks that the person with dementia may begin to find difficult, for example finances, paying bills and ensuring sufficient funds are transferred between bank accounts. However, if the diagnosis is made when the person living with dementia is later in their journey, some family members and partners may have already begun to assume more responsibility for activities of daily living, such as shopping and cooking, and also assist with personal care, for example dressing or bathing. Family members and friends can find themselves on a roller coaster that they try to valiantly navigate. The changes in the role may also occur gradually and slowly over time. It really all depends on how the individual with the diagnosis of dementia progresses and the issues that they find challenging (Senturk et al., 2018).

Family members report feelings of loss and sadness when they take on the care and support role. These can include:

> **Loss of intimacy and relationship** – Many spouse carers and child carers report experiencing a change in their relationship, that the previous closeness with the person with dementia changes and that they lose the person who perhaps provided them with support, be it emotional, practical or both (Youell et al., 2016; O'Shaughnessy et al., 2010; Quinn et al., 2009).
>
> **Loss of social opportunities** – Many care supporters, along with the person with dementia, find that they become socially isolated. After diagnosis the primary care supporter may avoid other family and friends because they do not know how to tell others or do not want others to know of the diagnosis. This may be due to feelings of guilt, shame or embarrassment, fear of how others may react and wanting to try and avoid others 'interfering' with the domestic situation. Social isolation may

lead to feelings of loneliness and being 'trapped' in a role or in a physical space that was previously a sanctuary, the home, with little opportunity for the care supporters to have time to themselves. Isolation can lead to a loss of self-confidence and contribute to low mood. The person with dementia may find it difficult to cope with social situations and no longer wish to leave the home or attend groups and functions they previously found enjoyable (Quinn et al., 2012). This can be a stressful experience for the spouse or adult child-care supporter of a person living with dementia if they feel they are pressuring the person with dementia to socialise.

Loss of relationships with other family members and friends – There may be conflict within a family or circle of friends. Family and friends may stop calling round to visit or may stop telephoning the family. Often this is because they do not have an understanding of dementia, do not know how to deal with the person or do not want to acknowledge changes in the person with dementia. It can be particularly difficult for the family supporter of the person with dementia to adjust to the loss of a vital support network at a time when they are sorely in need of additional support rather than less. Family conflict can also arise if family members, particularly children, disagree with the diagnosis and treatment plans, or if they deny the changes that are happening to the person with dementia due to their less intense exposure to the situation that the closest family members may have been masking for some time prior to the diagnosis.

Loss of confidence and motivation – Some family members describe a loss of confidence as they try to take on a role that they had not expected and are not prepared for (Shim et al., 2012). Low confidence whilst caring can lead to other problems such as depression or anxiety. Even after relinquishing their care and support role due to death or a move into long-term care, for example, family members, spouses and children can feel a lack of confidence in adjusting back to 'life' without the person with dementia by their side. Their whole life may gradually have evolved to revolve around meeting the person with dementia's needs and as a result they forgot about looking after their own needs.

Impact on mental and physical health – Those supporting people living with dementia have been reported as experiencing higher rates of depression and poorer physical health than those who do not provide care or support for a relative or friend. Rates of depression in care supporters of people with dementia can be high (Watson et al., 2019) and are a clear demonstration of the support people require.

There can be a role reversal for some when the spouse/partner develops dementia. For example:

Who manages the finances – Managing the finances and ensuring family expenses are covered may need to be handled by a new person. The person with dementia or their partner may have been the primary earner in the home, and if the person with dementia can no longer work, or the person required to provide support or care can no longer work, there can be a change in financial circumstances as income may be significantly reduced. The family as a whole may face financial hardship and experience worry about the ability to pay bills and rent or mortgage. Reduced income can also affect lifestyle, as less money might mean less social and/or transport opportunities and result in isolation for both the family care supporter and the person with dementia.

Who is responsible for driving – One of the more practical changes that a person with dementia is likely to experience is the transition from driver to passenger, and this may mean that the family supporter transitions from being the passenger to being the driver. While this may seem a logical transition as a result of increasing cognitive difficulties (particularly for driving authorities such as the Driver and Vehicle Licensing Agency or DVLA), it may represent a huge loss and be an emotionally difficult transition for both the person with dementia and their care supporter(s). In addition to the practical advantages of being a driver, driving may also be related to an individual's self-respect, social membership and independence (McKillop, 2016). The negative effects of the transition from driver to passenger extend beyond the person with dementia and often cause stress and emotional issues for the care partner too as they begin to take on the responsibility for driving to appointments, for shopping and to social engagements. This loss and transition may be the one that really brings home the diagnosis of dementia for all concerned.

FACTORS THAT INFLUENCE THE CARE SUPPORTER ROLE EXPERIENCE

Different factors may impact on the experience of providing care and support. We will first consider the evidence in relation to gender differences and then also discuss the potential impact of sexual orientation and ethnicity on the care and support experience. There are of course many other factors that will impact on the experience of caregiving and support, and although our discussion is limited to these three particular issues, the take-home message is to see the care supporter as an individual in their own right whose experiences of providing support and care will be shaped by a multitude of factors.

Gender differences

Those providing support to the person living with dementia are more likely to be female (whether they are employed to provide care or whether they are supporting a relative or friend who lives with dementia) (Alzheimer Disease International, 2015). Historically and traditionally,

- Centuries of socialisation means that women are often seen as 'natural' carers by others in the family.
- Women may marry older men and live longer themselves.
- Women's socio-economic positioning the family may lead to taking on caregiving roles.

Bamford and Walker (2012) demonstrate that globally women have and will continue to be those who are most impacted by dementia and that ongoing sex discrimination is likely to negatively impact on women. They argue that policy makers need to address this if future dementia care policy is to ensure positive outcomes for both those with the diagnosis and those providing support.

Sherman and Boss (2007), in a study of women's late life re-marriage and their experiences of dementia, revealed an interplay between complex family dynamics, particularly conflict within new and existing family members and profound experiences of loss and isolation. Despite this, the wife caregivers took proactive approaches to caring for their husbands, attributing their coping skills to their prior experiences of loss. Yet this also made them vulnerable to neglect by families and health and social care services, as their perceived coping competence obscured their need for help and support. This study also highlights that sometimes 'family-focused' interventions and support may be inappropriate, particularly in families experiencing negative family dynamics, and that support for the care supporters is key.

The primary difference reported in the literature between men and women providing care and support to their partner/spouse is that women appear to be more likely to experience stress than men (Gibbons et al., 2014). Strategies to alleviate stress have been suggested. For example, Blake et al. (2006) discuss the role of humour in caregiving and, although mainly relating it to formal caregivers, they advocate its use (where appropriate and when therapeutic) as a way of bridging the distance between the person with dementia and their care supporter. While research on the satisfactions of providing care support challenge dominant conceptualisations of caregiving where burden and stress are emphasised, Dartington's (2007) first-hand description shows that burden, stress and positive elements of caring are interwoven throughout the caring journey. Providing care and support is a demanding role that brings both satisfactions and challenges for the care supporter. Ensuring that the needs of the person providing care and support are met is an area that has been recognised by policy as important to address (Alzheimer Disease International, 2017) but one that is not always a reality.

Much research on those providing care neglected and marginalised the work and experiences of men; those that do include male caregivers often explored their experiences as a contrast to the experiences of women rather than focusing on their experiences first and foremost (Russell, 2008).

Levesque et al. (2008), in their study of older husband caregivers in Canada, found that men experienced stress brought on by changes in their marital relationship with their wives, but also that caring for their wives was a source of personal enrichment – by bolstering their usefulness. Similarly, Riberio and Paul (2008), in their study of elderly male caregivers who were looking after chronically ill wives, found that most of the men who were interviewed expressed at least one positive aspect to their care role. These included:

- Affirming their commitment to their marriage.
- New challenges.
- New purpose.
- New role.
- A sense of achievement in their caring.
- Sense of renewed self-esteem and self-worth.
- Knowledge that they provided a level of care that might not be provided by others.

Baker and Robertson's (2008) review of the literature of male and female spouse care supporters found inconclusive evidence as to differences between males and females. They suggest that there may be similarities in coping styles of those who are managing their caregiving role successfully. In a study exploring gender identity and perceptions of strain and burden, Baker et al. (2010) suggests that male caregivers with traditional beliefs about masculinity were more likely to say that

1 They are not feeling burdened.
2 They feel uncertain about caring.
3 They are more likely to articulate positive aspects to being a spousal carer than men with less traditional beliefs about masculinity.

In another review of male caregiving (Robinson et al., 2014), it was found that gendered identities and notions of masculinity were inherent in men's experiences of caring for a person living with dementia, in the way they understood and experienced relational factors and also on the reported outcomes for the men. This suggests that it is not gender per se that leads to differences in experiences but how the person providing support organises their understanding of their role in relation to their gendered identities. Rather than looking for gender differences Robinson et al. (2014) suggest that a better understanding of gender relations may enable greater insights into the experiences of providing care and support and how best to respond to the needs of care supporters that would have the best outcomes for their own physical and mental wellbeing. Using the example of cooking, Boyle (2013) demonstrates that men may refuse to cook, cook together or take over cooking when their partner develops dementia and that their approach largely demonstrates their traditional gendered relationship. In this way it is not that men cannot cook (although some may feel they cannot) but that the roles they take on when providing support relate to their identities as men and the relationship they have with their partner, both before and when their partner had dementia.

Bartlett et al. (2018) argue that the voices of men and women are going unheard in dementia care. This may be due to the way researchers, policy makers and practitioners may talk about caregiving generally without giving due consideration to the impact of gender and gendered identities and the resultant norms and expectations on experiences of providing support and care (and also the experience of living with dementia). Yet the research clearly demonstrates that the gendered identities of individual care supporters may influence their caregiving experiences and their perceived abilities to cope with the demands of their roles.

Experience of gay, lesbian, bisexual and transgender care supporters

The literature discussed so far focuses on heterosexual couples living within traditional family structures. Of course this will not be representative of the families of all people with dementia. Relatively little is known about the experiences of gay and lesbian couples and how they adapt and cope following a diagnosis of dementia. Most carer support services and groups are based on a traditional model of a family with the main care supporter being a wife or daughter. This is changing as noted above with acknowledgement of the increasingly important role of male carers. However, there is still relatively little acknowledgment of the experiences and needs of lesbian and gay carers. Westwoods' (2016) recent edited collection *Lesbian, Gay, Bisexual and Trans* Individuals Living with Dementia: Concepts, Practice and Rights* provides a much-needed overview of the experiences and issues affecting carers, as well as people living with dementia, who identify as non-heterosexual.

Newman (2005) provided an early account of his experiences of caring for his partner, who was diagnosed with dementia at the age of 56. Newman (2005) describes himself as a 'joiner' whose natural response to the diagnosis was to join the Alzheimer's Society in England and to attend carers' groups. He found, however, that he was not able to identify with the other carers and that magazines and other literature seemed to assume that dementia only 'affected married couples or those with supportive families' (Newman, 2005, 266). In response to his experiences, Newman began to search for other gay and lesbian carers and his work led to the development of a specialist Lesbian, Gay, Bisexual and Transgender Support Group. There is now an increasing movement to ensure the needs and rights of LGBTQ people are recognised. Mike Parish provides an account of the satisfactions and frustrations in providing care to his husband Tom (2017), highlighting the change that has occurred since 2005 when Newman felt completely isolated.

Research in this area has been developing a pace. In the UK, Price (2010) examined the experiences of a sample of gay men and lesbian woman providing care to their partners with dementia. She describes her participant group as 'highly educated, politically informed and active, mainly urban dwelling individuals who were, on the whole, confident with their sexuality and willing to challenge oppressive practices' (Price, 2010, 167). Despite this their experiences of care services varied from acceptance at best and a lack of acknowledgement of their support needs at worst. She concluded that service providers need to review their attitudes towards sexuality. Similarly in Australia, Barrett et al.'s (2015) research with LGBT participants found that people were often isolated and left unsupported due to the responses they had received, or perceived they would receive from service providers. They argue that, 'aged care service providers need to better understand the experiences and needs of LGBT people living with dementia and advocate to ensure that dementia is not a barrier to expression of sexual orientation and gender' (Barrett et al., 2015, 37). Campaigns to raise awareness of the need to recognise the rights and support needs of LGBQT carers have led to an increased recognition of their needs, but the impact on experiences of services is less clear. A useful resource has been compiled by the UK Alzheimer Society that provides a starting point of issues to consider and can be found at www.alzheimers.org.uk/get-support/help-dementia-care/lgbt-dementia-care-other-resources.

Experiences of different cultural and ethnic groups

Much of the early work on race and ethnicity in dementia care came from the US (Dilworth-Anderson et al., 2002). Early reviews seeking to explore the experiences of different cultural and ethnic groups (Daker-White et al., 2002) found that people from minority ethnic groups are less likely to seek help for concerns relating to dementia symptoms. There was a lack of consensus in the literature as to whether specific services targeting minority ethnic communities were required or whether mainstream services would be sufficient (Daker-White et al., 2002); but what was clear was that there was a lack of specialist knowledge about the needs of ethnic groups and a corresponding lack of appropriate services (Beattie et al., 2005).

There has often been an assumption that ethnic groups wish to 'care for their own', however research examining this conception has found that people experiencing ethnic-related disadvantage actually wished to find support to enable them to relinquish additional stress and strain brought about by providing care to the person living with dementia (Gelman et al., 2014). This demonstrates a need to provide services and support that meet the needs of family members who may have entered into caregiving reluctantly and who would actively seek help if the opportunities were made available, as they were in Gelman et al.'s (2014) New York–based programme to support carers from minority groups, wo argue that

> despite popular and professional assumptions that ethnic minority families are able and willing to provide care to their older members, and may, in fact, prefer to do so rather than rely on formal care, this may be increasingly less the case for many families, and alternatives must be provided.
>
> (Gelman et al., 2014, 679)

The role of cultural values in societies, rather than ethnicity per se, has been convincingly argued to be of key importance when it comes to understanding the way different groups may understand care, how they experience stress and strain and the types of support and services they may need (Knight and Sayegh, 2010). Culture acknowledges the multitude of factors that may influence the experiences of caregiving beyond a simple ethnic categorisation. This is important, as the experiences of ethnic groups are diverse and the interconnections between ethnicity, age, gender, health status and so on are complex and therefore it is not solely 'ethnicity' that will impact on the experiences of caregiving. In their edited collection, Botsford and Dening (2015) provide us with examples of when individuals who experience cultural and language differences are isolated but they also provide examples of where culture is a source of support; as such their book provides a good overview of the challenges facing practitioners and communities and individuals when seeking to understand and support caregivers from culturally and ethnically diverse groups.

The differences and similarities in the experiences of people from different cultural and ethnic groups has been investigated, with US research finding that African Americans reported less stress than Caucasian Americans; the author links this to income and psychological resourcefulness, with the African American samples reporting higher levels of psychological resourcefulness than their more wealthy Caucasian counterparts (Bekhet, 2015). Recent research (Richardson et al., 2019) found that the stress and strain experienced by caregivers was pervasive across the three different ethnic groups (African American, Hispanic and South Korean); however cultural differences also existed with different levels of knowledge about dementia, language barriers, religion and spirituality and cultural differences in attitudes about caring and formal services all influencing the caregiving experience.

Research exploring the impact of ethnic and cultural groups provides us with insights into the needs of different groups, but the key similarity is that all individuals providing care may need support.

EXPERIENCES OF PROVIDING CARE AND SUPPORT: 'SATISFACTION' AND 'BURDEN'

Regardless of the gender, ethnicity or other characteristics of the person providing support and care, it is common to hear people talk about the burden and stress of caring. But how real is this 'burden' and 'stress'?

Ho et al. (2009) explored the impact of caregiving on health and quality of life among Asian families who practiced filial piety (that is, being good to/looking after ones parents). They found that caregivers had significantly increased risks for reporting worse health, more doctor's visits, anxiety and depression, and weight loss (2009, 873). They found that females were more likely to report sleeping disorders, chronic diseases, symptoms and insomnia. In their recent European study, Janssen et al. (2017) found that caregiver profiles could be created based on demographic factors and their coping styles and abilities and that a combination of factors was important to alleviate depression and feelings of burden and to promote wellbeing and quality of life amongst caregivers of people living with dementia. They specifically linked the age of the care supporter in relation to the degree of strain experienced. While the level of strain experienced could still be variable, age was a factor. There is also evidence that family members experience physical and psychological stress as a direct result of how they manage their own health and needs with the responsibilities of providing support and care (McCabe et al., 2016).

Research indicates there may be gender differences in caregiving burden and abilities to handle acute or chronic stress when providing care and support, yet the picture is far from clear and demonstrates the complexities in providing care and support to a person living with dementia. For example, one study by Mills et al. (2009) found that being a male carer for a spouse with severe dementia is associated with increased risk of sleep disturbance and cardiovascular disease. One explanation for this might be that the carer role is more culturally associated with females than males.

There is substantial evidence to suggest that female carers experience more strain than male carers, with increased levels of depression and lowered morale. Assumptions that all care supporters are stressed can fail to take account of the differences in coping skills, personality and individual appraisal systems, which all impact on the experience of caring (Quinn et al., 2012). Knussen et al. (2008) found that care supporters who increased the proportion of strategies to maintain 'balance' between caregiving and other personal interests experienced less distress. Their study highlights the potential benefits to carers of maintaining a balance in their lives by taking regular breaks from providing support.

Farfan-Portet et al. (2009) identify that caregiver burden for informal carers, compared with non-caregivers, is subjectively worse in terms of health, depression, adopting riskier health behaviours, poorer immune systems and higher risk of death. There is also a relationship between the amount of time caring and the impact on the caregiver's health, with more weekly hours of caring being associated with increased risk of poor health (Farfan-Portet et al., 2009). Carers of working age face different issues; when they do manage to balance both work and caring commitments, they are often faced with continued disadvantage. They may work below their skill level, have a reduced likelihood of promotion and earn less than their non-carer counterparts. They report having to take more time off than colleagues and often use holiday entitlement to cover their caring role (Ramcharan and Whittell, 2003). Establishing or reawakening sources of satisfaction in carers of people with dementia could enable the development of services that focus on areas of strengths and expertise and acknowledge that rewards and satisfactions co-exist with stress in the lives of many carers.

The concept of how to help build resilience in care supporters has received increased attention (Senturk et al., 2018; Bekhet and Avery, 2018; Dias et al., 2015; Donnellan et al., 2015). By providing opportunities for care supporters to learn more about dementia, talk to others in similar situations and to have time to ensure their own interests and physical health needs are met are all factors that can contribute to care supporters being able to continue to support the person living with dementia and to derive satisfaction from doing so. Jenssen et al.'s (2017) European study demonstrates the complexities of the factors that lead to stress in different types of caregivers according to age, relationship to the person with dementia (which includes gender), how severe the dementia may be and the ways individuals adapt to stress. This all demonstrates that differences in experiences are multi-faceted and complex with no simple explanation as to who may or may not experience stress or strain and at particular moments in time.

Experiences of caring for someone with dementia

The website link below is a short film of the experiences of one man who cares for his wife who has dementia and who continues to live at home.

SCIE (2009) Rapidly Declining Early-Onset Dementia: Living at Home with Nursing Support www.scie.org.uk/dementia/carers-of-people-with-dementia//supporting-carers/early-onset-living-at-home-with-nursing-support.asp

CHALLENGES WHEN PROVIDING SUPPORT TO A PERSON LIVING WITH DEMENTIA

Behaviour is an important form of social conduct and also of non-verbal communication. It can be an expression of boredom, loneliness, pain, fear, self-identity or just a way of saying 'I don't like what you are doing to me' or 'I don't like where I am'. For the person with dementia, different behaviours are often reactions or responses to internal or external stimuli, and importantly all behaviour has meaning – the difficulty can be working out what the meaning is. How the person interprets this information and their reality is crucially dependent on their physiological/neurological impairment and the social and built environment (Kitwood, 1997).

McCabe et al. (2016) review of the expressed needs of care supporters found that those providing support needed help to manage the needs of the person living with dementia, for example how to assist with activities of daily living, how to cope with some of the commonly associated behavioural symptoms of dementia and how to access both formal services to help them cope with their role and other forms of informal support, such as peer support from others providing a care or support role to family members.

There are many strategies, some simple and some requiring more effort, that care supporters can use to help them cope with situations they find difficult. These include:

- Removing (if safe to do so for both the care supporter and the person living with dementia) themselves from the situation.
- Learning certain biological triggers for certain behaviours that may be difficult for the care supporter to respond to (pain, hunger, constipation) and developing strategies to either minimise the chance of these occurring (e.g. for those listed here this may be regular pain relief, ensuring snacks are available, a fibre-rich diet).
- Learning about the psychological triggers (fear, anxiety, boredom, frustration) that may lead to the difficulties in interacting with the person living with dementia, and again having strategies to minimise the risk of these occurring and ways to respond that the person finds helpful if they do.
- Reducing sensory triggers (noise, bright light, too warm, too cold).

Intimacy, sexuality and sexual behaviour

The need for touch, intimacy and sex remain important in the lives of older people and people with dementia (Youell et al., 2016). Evans and Lee's (2014) review of the impact on the marriage of people living with dementia demonstrates the difficulties in retaining a sense of intimacy; as care needs progress to physical and personal care, sex and physical intimacy can become problematic. In research exploring women's experiences of caring for men with dementia, participants reported missing the lack of affection and attention that they experienced as the dementia progressed and their relationship with their spouse changed (Walters et al., 2010). Men have also reported feeling a loss of intimacy as they begin to do physical care for the person living with dementia (Harris, 2009), demonstrating that this is something experienced by men and women. Continual intimacy and sexual activity is most often a factor of adjustment for the caregivers of people with dementia who are married or long-term partners.

There has been a limited focus on sexuality and sexual behaviour for people with dementia and their partners/spouses. However, research on this area is increasing in recognition of its importance. Studies have shown that providing information about sexuality and dementia and a psycho-behavioural approach can decrease the strain of families and care supporters (Lipinska, 2017; Ward et al., 2005). Although intimacy, including sexual intimacy, remains an important element of older couple relationships, expressing needs and maintaining this form of connection was at times difficult for participants (Youell et al., 2016). Retaining relationships is important for both people living with dementia and their partners and family members. In chapter 5 we will consider how to address the combined support needs of people with dementia and their partners/family members.

SUPPORT SERVICES FOR THOSE PROVIDING CARE AND SUPPORT

Studies of the service use of care supporters of people living with dementia are relatively rare. Martindale-Adams et al. (2016) found that a variety of factors led to increased service use by those providing support to a person living with dementia. Those who were older, more educated, married, not employed, depressed, used more medications, had more symptoms and spent fewer hours on duty per day used significantly more services for themselves. Higher service use indicated greater burden, difficulty in dealing with behaviours of the person with dementia, and more desire to institutionalise.

Providing respite for the care supporter to enable them to have regular breaks from their role has received much attention, as Neville et al.'s (2015) review demonstrates. However, trying to work out exactly what might work in the way of respite provision and under what circumstances is difficult. The review authors suggest that when respite is provided at the point where the care supporter is finding it increasingly difficult, the impact or outcomes may be less than if support was provided at an earlier point facilitating the person providing support to continue to do so for longer.

It is important that those providing support and care have access to support themselves, but anecdotally, we hear all too often of people who really want to support the person living with dementia but who also need some support that they cannot access for whatever reason. Innes et al.'s (2011) review of informal caregivers in rural areas demonstrates the multitude of factors that can compound the geographic remoteness and isolation in providing support to the person living with dementia.

In this chapter, we have looked in more detail at what the experiences of being a care supporter for a person living with dementia may involve. We have looked at some of the losses that may be experienced by care supporters and some of the things that may lead to different experiences of those providing the support role. The relationship between the care supporter and the person living with dementia also affects this experience.

We have looked at some of the differences experienced by care supporters that have been reported in the literature. For example, the experiences of men and women, people from different ethnic groups and people from the LGBTQ community. All of these examples demonstrate that the experience of providing support and care can be as different for each individual care supporter as the uniqueness of each individual living with dementia. Person-centred care is not just about recognising the individuality of the person with dementia, it is also about recognising the individuality of each person providing care and how their experiences of this role are complex and shaped and influenced by a variety of characteristics and the responses of others to these characteristics.

The account below written by Gail, in her own words, about her experiences of her mother's post-diagnostic journey, her father's post-diagnostic journey and her personal reflections on her caregiving role provide a clear account of how many different issues impact on the experience of providing support.

Gerry Bowkers' story as told by her daughter Gail

When given my mum's diagnosis of dementia I was angry at the way the meeting was going and felt somehow let down by the process, so I asked to meet with the doctor at a time more convenient. She sighed then agreed to meet the following week. That encounter began my turbulent and sometimes quite fractious dealings with the Memory Assessment and Treatment Team (MATs) and the NHS as a whole.

There were very few groups or organisations that mum, dad and I could have benefited from. Mum didn't like noise, was fearful of hospital-looking buildings and only felt comfortable at home. There were no home therapy sessions on offer nor were there any admiral nurses to obtain support and advice from. Technically we were all alone. As a carer I had no support and found that I was feeling more frustrated with this.

District nurses eventually became involved and at one point the GP called in a rapid response team following his parting comment to me that I 'really have no alternative but to have mum put into a nursing home'. This was a nightmare from beginning to end. Mum had deteriorated slightly due to a urinary tract infection. She refused to get out of bed and any notion of going downstairs was quickly dismissed. She became paranoid and suspicious of everything and everyone and started to hallucinate. When the rapid response team arrived the way dad and I were treated was tantamount to bullying. I was not listened to – anything I said was either ignored or skirted over and I was told that the bed had to go, to be replaced with a hospital style one. The bed had been a wedding present to my parents and had a lot of sentimentality attached. When I said 'no' I was quickly told that I was putting sentimentality over the welfare of my mum, to which I replied 'I am putting the thoughts and feelings of my father in as much context as the welfare of my mother. I am seeing the whole picture not the tunnel vision view you have'. Perseverance on my part saw a compromise being reached which resulted in mum being moved into my bedroom and me sleeping on the floor. Eventually I bought a fold-up bed – I put it away every morning and brought it out again every evening. This was my routine for the next few years. Everyday became an uphill struggle with the NHS, National Institute for Health and Care Excellence (NICE), the Clinical Commissioning Group (CCG) and the Memory Assessment Treatment Team (MATs). I had to fight for everything – drugs, support, equipment, incontinence pads and for professionals to listen. I was only a carer, so what did I know! The 'closed doors' I encountered of the CCG and the GP saw me having to involve my local member of Parliament (MP) in a battle over medication. As mum found tablets hard to swallow she required a liquid version. As this cost more money, mum was refused the treatment. Once the MP intervened, the medication was allowed. The CCG had felt that mum would not have benefited, but how wrong they were. Her hallucinations became less frequent and she became calm, enough to improve her quality of life. She began to enjoy music again, having her cousin visit and her relationship with dad and I was as it had been before.

There was one professional angel in this journey, mum's community psychiatric nurse (CPN). Mel was there through thick and thin. She supported us not only practically, but emotionally too, becoming a friend. Mum looked forward to Mel's visits – Mel would kneel beside mum, holding her hand, and would talk to her about everything – the weather, the news, what soft toy mum was nursing that day and most of all treated mum with dignity and respect. She even sat with mum if I had to take dad to a hospital appointment. Her friendship remains with us today. Eventually we were put in contact with the local hospice that had a hospice-at-home team. After an assessment they agreed to offer respite sits once a week so I could take dad out for the afternoon. These became invaluable as it allowed us time to reflect but also to breathe.

The one thing that was evident: dementia was always the first condition the professionals would see. Mum started to have recurring chest infections. Doctors were quick to say that she was aspirating due to problems with swallowing brought on by her dementia. However, one trainee GP came to see mum and felt that there was more to the infections, especially when her leg began to swell. He arranged for an emergency scan at a clinic; he even arranged the transport. The GP also made sure that a consultant saw mum following the scan. His concerns were confirmed: mum had cancer. Due to the severity of her dementia, mum was refused cancer treatment under NICE guidance. Instead she was offered palliative treatment, which technically meant I had to administer Oramorph when she was in pain. I approached MacMillan Cancer Support and even they said there was nothing they could offer to us as a family. Their rationale was that district nurses were involved and they were not trained for dementia. Mum lived for 18 months following the diagnosis of cancer.

As a carer but ultimately as a daughter I felt quite let down the way mum was treated following her diagnosis of dementia. As a family we became emotionally drained with the constant battles. But the one person who was completely failed by the system was mum.

Ron Bowkers' story as told by his daughter Gail

Once dad had received the diagnosis, a support worker from the Memory Assessment Team came to the house to see what support if any we required; again a refreshing change from my experience with my mother before. Also, Mel, mum's community psychiatric nurse (CPN), was assigned to dad, so I knew we had one friend through dad's dementia journey.

As dad has a vascular dementia the only medication he was prescribed was medicine he was already taking following a stroke in 2002. One thing I have noticed is that unless a person takes some form of dementia medication then there is no follow up from the Memory Assessment Team. This follow up is normally an appointment with a psychiatrist to monitor the medication and to make amendments as required. If the person is not on any of the medications, then the aftercare is pushed back to the GP, who should monitor the progression. This is still to happen!

Non-medical support has continued for dad and I since mum passed away. I researched different groups that I thought dad might be interested in, and the main place that he actually enjoys being is at the Salford Institute for Dementia (Salford University). Here he enjoys music therapy sessions, being involved with research and being part of something where he feels valued. He once said that he 'felt wanted' – this sense of belonging is vitally important for dad. He had quite a fractious relationship with his own family and never felt 'wanted' – so his vulnerability with dementia coupled with other health issues and memories of his childhood mean that he needs to have that feeling of belonging. We have tried other groups for him, but it is sometimes difficult to enter groups of existing members, and so where this occurs, he never felt comfortable – so we avoid these.

Dad also has the opportunity to talk about his varied career – from being a musician, a grocer, a tea blender, a postman and when he joined the St John Ambulance as a first responder. It is important that he can still relate to his identity of being someone who has a passion for music but who can also save lives. He is fiercely proud of this and proudly wears his silver badge for valued service.

The one thing post-diagnostically for dad is that he still has the ability to communicate, can remember events, but equally does not consider that he has dementia. I have been angered by some professionals who correct him when he says he does not have dementia, as in his mind he is still the same person as he always was. He also doesn't relate to dementia as his main experience was with mum – and as he doesn't present with the same symptoms, he therefore doesn't think he has the disease. When professionals talk about his condition in front of him, he becomes slightly distressed, even though I have often asked that they refrain from mentioning the word dementia.

What does upset me is that some of dad's closest friends stopped calling round to see him. The reason was that they felt that they might upset him, or may not be able to communicate with him. But thankfully dad has made new friends within the dementia community. As he is a sociable person, and a bit of a flirt with the ladies – it makes him feel alive!

There are still issues within the professional arena regarding dementia. Especially the fact that dementia is still the first condition seen, which means that other illnesses can be missed. I still have to push doctors to see beyond the dementia, particularly when he is hospitalised for other conditions. Dad had a severe reaction to an antibiotic which resulted in him developing epilepsy. One doctor said that the seizures were a result of the dementia, but with further investigation it was agreed that the seizures were due to the medication.

Our journey is still continuing and dad is still able to have a quality of life. He lives every day to its fullest and reminds me that he is still my dad!

Gail's story of providing care and support to her parents

My name is Gail and I am a carer, or at least that's what the label says! It all began nine years ago when I embarked on a new journey within the chapters of my life. It was the journey of dementia.

An author named Rosie Staal wrote a poignant book, *What Shall We Do with Mother?*, that described various peoples' journeys as care providers. The following piece started me on my rollercoaster ride post-diagnostic; a ride that took me through the trials and tribulations I was to encounter as I entered into the frightening and lonely place being a care provider can take you:

> Stepping up a gear in middle age to accommodate the needs of an ageing parent involves both physical and mental adjustment. Life will never be the same again when you take on the responsibility of someone else's welfare, but neither is it likely to be dull and uneventful.

The author was not wrong. I found that undertaking this role certainly had the label attached – *carer*. No longer was I a daughter, I was just a carer. I became invisible, and to make things worse some family friends shied away – frightened of the word *dementia*, and feeling uncomfortable to even talk about it. Some would say that they didn't know how to speak to mum and dad, or others would say that they wanted to remember them how they were pre-dementia. This was their loss!

When I first became a care partner I was still working full time, and my job was my only respite, but even this became difficult to maintain. Juggling full-time caring roles for two people with a full-time job took its toll both physically and emotionally. As an only child with no other immediate family other than one cousin and mum's elderly cousins, all the responsibility fell to me.

I had decided that I would look after mum and dad myself at home. What I found at the beginning was the lack of support offered to the person with dementia but more so carers. It was a case of 'just get on with it'. I wasn't made aware of any benefits that I might be entitled to, nor was I made aware until several years later that I should have had a carers' assessment. This assessment looks at what your needs are to allow you to undertake your caring role. By the time I had been assessed I had already resigned from my job, had paid for carers to come in for a couple of hours a day until I finished work and I had made numerous telephone calls to various government departments to see if we as a family qualified for any benefits. I just got on with it as I was told to, but it did have some consequences.

I felt alone, isolated and on many an occasion I would sit on the kitchen floor a blubbering wreck asking the same question – WHY?

Why did mum have to develop dementia with Lewy bodies, why did dad five years later develop vascular dementia? I felt that I had no support other than from Mel, the community psychiatric nurse, my dear friend Julie and my wonderful neighbours. Interestingly, professional support was nonexistent other than Mel.

Whilst still working the only support I had came from my team – my second family, but this support ended with them. My senior officers were not sympathetic to my circumstances, especially when I applied for a career break and was only offered four months. So, it was the easiest decision to make: resign. Mum and dad were more important, but by resigning I also isolated myself even further.

Mum was at a stage where she would not leave the house, which meant that dad and I stayed in also. The furthest I travelled was to the local shops or to the hospital with dad. This was until I was put in touch with the hospice-at-home team who offered one afternoon per week as respite. They would stay with mum, whilst dad and I could go out. It doesn't sound much, but when you are suffering from cabin fever you take what you can get!

My support only came when mum had passed away in 2017. Dad and I were now able to seek groups that we could go to. This was an epiphany for me as a whole new world opened up. I met some amazing people within the dementia groups and these are now my new dementia family. The support I was seeking for so many years was now available and from this I have now embarked on a new journey. This journey is to address the inconsistency of support for all people going through post-diagnosis. I am now part of a movement for change, and best thing is I AM NOT ALONE.

Strangely if this disease had not come into my life, I would not have made the choices I did and therefore would not have had the chance to make such wonderful memories with mum and dad. I want to use my experiences and skill sets to enrich other people's lives, so they do not have to go through the same frustrations I have endured. And, most of all I want to highlight that carers are not a label – we are articulate, educated professionals with a vast array of knowledge to impart. We have experience, we need support and most of all we need to be listened to. The carer is the wealth of knowledge about the person they care for, from past medical history to common routines. Without these details the professionals would struggle. We therefore need to work together so we can attain the same goal – the welfare of the person living with dementia. Unfortunately, I believe that much is yet to be done in this field as I have witnessed firsthand the 'malignant social psychology' within the professional arena from district nurses, hospitals and care homes. I must say that we do have a fabulous district nurse who seems to understand dementia, but she is one out of many others who don't.

I want professionals and others to see me for who I am – a daughter first and foremost, but a person like them who just happens to be a carer; who needs support, guidance and friendship throughout the dementia ride; and most of all wants to be respected for the contributions I am making to society by undertaking my caring role.

There are many online resources with tips and ideas for how care supporters can look after themselves and how they can support the person living with dementia at home for as long as possible. Here are some that we think are particularly useful.

Resources for those providing care

Alzheimer Society www.alzheimers.org.uk/get-support/help-dementia-care/caring-for-person-dementia#content-start

Alzheimer Canada https://alzheimer.ca/en/Home/Living-with-dementia/Caring-for-someone

Dementia Action Alliance www.dementiaaction.org.uk/carers/examples_of_services_and_support

Dementia UK www.dementiauk.org/sources-of-support-for-families/

National Institute for Health and Care Excellence www.nice.org.uk/about/nice-communities/social-care/tailored-resources/dementia

NHS Health Scotland www.healthscotland.scot/health-topics/dementia

REFERENCES

Alzheimer's Disease International (2015) *Women and Dementia: A Global Research Review*. London: Alzheimer's Disease International.

Alzheimer's Disease International (2017) *National Dementia Action Plans: Examples for Inspiration*. Swiss Federal Office of Public Health.

www.alz.co.uk/sites/default/files/pdfs/national-plans-examples-2017.pdf

Baker, K.L. and Robertson, N. (2008) Coping with caring for someone with dementia: Reviewing the literature about men. *Aging andMental Health* 12(4):413–422.

Baker, K.L., Robertson, N. and Connelly, D. (2010) Men caring for wives or partners with dementia: Masculinity, strain and gain. *Aging andMental Health* 14(3):319–327.

Bamford, S.M. and Walker, T. (2012) Women and dementia: Not forgotten. *Maturitas* 73(2):121–126.

Barrett, C., Crameri, P., Lambourne, S., Latham, J.R. and Whyte, C. (2015) Understanding the experiences and needs of lesbian, gay, bisexual and trans Australians living with dementia, and their partners. *Australasian Journal on Aging* 34(2):34–38. Doi: 10.1111/ajag.12271

Bartlett, R., Gjernes, T., Lotherington, A. and Obstefelder, A. (2018) Gender, citizenship and dementia care: A scoping review of studies to inform policy and future research. *Health and Social Care in the Community* 26(1):14–26. https://doi.org/10.1111/hsc.12340

Beattie, B., Daker-White, G., Gilliard, J. and Means, R. (2005) They don't quite fit the way we organise our services': Results from a UK field study of marginalised groups and dementia care. *Disability and Society* 20(1):67–80.

Bekhet, A.K. (2015) Resourcefulness in African American and Caucasian American caregivers of persons with dementia: Associations with perceived burden, depression, anxiety, positive cognitions, and psychological well-being. *Perspectives in Psychiatric Care* 51:285–294.

Bekhet, A.K. and Avery, J.S. (2018) Resilience from the perspectives of caregivers of persons with dementia. *Archives of Psychiatric Nursing* 32(1):19–23.

Blake, W., Mills, M. and Coleman, P. (2006) The role of humour in dementia. In Miesen, B. and Jones, G. (Eds.), Care-Giving in Dementia: Research and Applications (Vol. 4). London: Routledge.

Botsford, J. and Dening, K.H. (eds.) (2015) *Dementia, Culture and Ethnicity: Issues for All.* London: Jessica Kingsley Publishers.

Boyle, G. (2013) "Can't cook, won't cook": Men's involvement in cooking when their wives develop dementia. *Journal of Gender Studies* 23(4):336–350.

Daker-White, G., Beattie, A.M., Gilliard, J. and Means, R. (2002) Minority ethnic groups in dementia care: A review of service needs, service provision and models of good practice. *Aging and Mental Health* 6(2):101–108. https://doi-org.salford.idm.oclc.org/10.1080/13607860220126835

Dartington, T. (2007). Two days in December. *Dementia* 6(3):327–341. https://doi.org/10.1177/1471301207081564

Dias, R., Santos, R.L., de Sousa, M.F., Nogueira, M.M., Torres, B. and Belfort, T. (2015) Resilience of caregivers of people with dementia: A systematic review of biological and psychosocial determinants. *Trends in Psychiatry and Psychotheraphy* 37(1):12–19.

Dilworth-Anderson, P., Williams, I.C. and Gibson, B.E. (2002) Issues of race, ethnicity, and culture in caregiving research: A 20-year review (1980–2000). *The Gerontologist* 42:237–272.

Donnellan, W.J., Bennett, K.M. and Soulsby, L.K. (2015) What are the factors that facilitate or hinder resilience in older spousal dementia carers? A qualitative study. *Aging and Mental Health* 19:932–939.

Evans, D. and Lee, E. (2014) Impact of dementia on marriage: A qualitative systematic review. *Dementia* 13(3):330–349. Doi: 10.1177/1471301212473882

Farfan-Portet, M., Popham, F., Mitchell, R., Swine, C. and Lorant, V. (2009) Caring, employment and health among adults of working age: Evidence from Britain and Belgium. *European Journal of Public Health*:1–6.

Gelman, C.R., Sokoloff, T., Graziani, N., Arias, E. And Peralta, A. (2014) Individually-tailored support for ethnically-diverse caregivers: Enhancing our understanding of what is needed and what works. *Journal of Gerontological Social Work* 57:662–680.

Gibbons, C., Creese, J., Tran, M., Brazil, K., Chambers, L., Weaver, B. and Bédard, M. (2014) The psychological and health consequences of caring for a spouse with dementia: A critical comparison of husbands and wives. *Journal of Women and Aging* 26(1):3–21.

Harris, P. (2009) Intimacy, sexuality and early-stage dementia: The changing marital relationship. *Alzheimer's Care Today* 10(2):63–77.

Ho, S., Chan, A., Woo, J., Chong, P. and Sham, A. (2009) Impact of caregiving on health and quality of life: A comparative population-based study of caregivers for elderly persons and noncaregivers. *Journal of Gerontology: Medical Sciences* 64A(8):873–879.

Innes, A., Morgan, D. and Kostenieuk, J. (2011) Informal dementia care in rural and remote settings: A systematic review. *Maturitas* 68(1):34–46.

Janssen, E.P., de Vugt, M., Köhler, S., Wolfs, C., Kerpershoek, L., Handels, R.L., Orrell, M., Woods, B., Jelley, H., Stephan, A., Bieber, A., Meyer, G., Engedal, K., Selbaek, G., Wimo, A., Irving, K., Hopper, L., Gonçalves-Pereira, M., Portolani, E., Zanetti, O. and Verhey, F.R. (2017) Caregiver profiles in dementia related to quality of life, depression and perseverance time in the European Actifcare study: The importance of social health. *Aging Mental Health* 21(1):49–57. Doi: 10.1080/13607863.2016.1255716

Kitwood, T. (1997) *Dementia Reconsidered: The Person Comes First.* Buckingham: Open University Press.

Knight, B.G. and Sayegh, P. (2010) Cultural values and caregiving: The updated sociocultural stress and coping model. *Journal of Gerontology: Psychological Sciences* 65B:5–13.

Knussen, C., Tolson, D., Brogan, C.A., Swan, I.R.C., Stott, D.J. and Sullivan, F. (2008) Family caregivers of older relatives: Ways of coping and change in distress. *Psychology, Health & Medicine* 13(3):274–290. doi: 10.1080/13548500701405483

Levesque, L., Ducharme, F., Zarit, S., Lachance, L. and Giroux, F. (2008) Predicting longitudinal patterns of psychological distress in older husband caregivers: Further analysis of existing data. *Aging and Mental Health* 12(3):333–342.

Lipinska, D. (2017) *Dementia, Sex and Wellbeing: A Person-Centred Guide for People with Dementia, Their Partners, Caregivers and Professionals.* London: Jessica Kingsley.

Martindale-Adams, J., Nichols, L.O., Zuber, J., Burns, R. and Graney, M.J. (2016) Dementia caregivers' user of services for themselves. *Gerontologist*:9. Doi: 10.1093/geront/gnv121

McCabe, M., You, E. and Tatangelo, G. (2016) Hearing their voice: A systematic review of dementia family caregivers' needs. *Gerontologist* 56(5):70–88.

McKillop, J. (2016) *Driving and Dementia: My Experiences.* Glasgow: Life Changes Trust. www.lifechangestrust.org.uk/sites/default/files/Driving%20with%20Dementia%20website.pdf

Mills, P. J., Ancoli-Israel, S., von Känel, R., Mausbach, B. T., Aschbacher, K., Patterson, T. L., Ziegler, M. G., Dimsdale, J. E. and Grant, I. (2009) Effects of gender and dementia severity on

Alzheimer's disease caregivers' sleep and biomarkers of coagulation and inflammation. *Brain, Behavior, and Immunity* 23(5):605–610. doi.org/10.1016/j.bbi.2008.09.014

Neville, C., Beattie, E., Fielding, E. and MacAndrew, M. (2015) Literature review: Use of respite by carers of people with dementia. *Health and Social Care in the Community* 23:51–64. Doi: edsgcl.397741909

Newman, R. (2005) Partners in care, neing equally different: Lesbian and gay carers. *Psychiatric Bulletin* 29:266–267.

O'Shaughnessey, M., Lee, K. and Lintern, T. (2010) Changes in couple relationship in dementia care: Spouse carers' experiences. Dementia 9(2):237–258.

Parish, M. (2017) Step into the light. *Dementia Together Magazine* December 17/January 18. www.alzheimers.org.uk/dementia-together-magazine/dec-jan-2017-2018/step-light

Price, E. (2010) Coming out to care: Gay and lesbian carers' experiences of dementia *services*. *Health and Social Care in the Community* 18(2):160–168. Doi: 10.1111/j.1365-2524.2009.00884.x

Quinn, C., Clare, L. and Woods, B. (2009) The impact of the quality of relationship on the experiences and wellbeing of caregivers of people with dementia: A systematic review. Aging andMental Health 13(2):143–154.

Quinn, C., Clare, L. and Woods, R.T. (2012) What predicts whether caregivers of people with dementia find meaning in their role? *International Journal of Geriatric Psychiatry* 27:1195–1202.

Ramcharan, P. and Whittell, B. (2003) Carers and employment. In Stalker, K. (Ed.), *Reconceptualising Work with 'Carers'. New Directions for Policy and Practice* (137–159). London: Jessica Kingsley Publishers.

Riberio, O. and Paul, C. (2008) Older male carers and the positive aspects of care. *Ageing and Society* 28:165–183.

Richardson, V.E., Fields, N., Daegu, S.W., Bradley, E., Gibson, A., Rivera, G. and Holmes, S.D. (2019) At the intersection of culture: Ethnically diverse dementia caregivers' service use. *Dementia* 18(5):1790–1809. Doi: 10.1177/147130121772130

Robinson, C.A., Bottorff, J.L., Pesut, B., Oliffe, J.L. and Tomlinson, J. (2014) The male face of caregiving: A scoping review of men caring for a person with dementia. *American Journal of Men's Health* 8(5):409–426.

Robinson, L., Clare, L. and Evans, K. (2005) Making sense of dementia and adjusting to loss: Psychological reactions to a diagnosis of dementia in couples. *Aging and Mental Health* 9(4):337–347.

Russell, R. (2008) Their story, my story: Health of older men as caregivers. *Generations*, Spring:62–67.

Senturk, S.G., Akyol, M.A. and Kucukguclu, O. (2018) The relationship between caregiver burden and psychological resilience in caregivers of individuals with dementia. *International Journal of Caring Sciences* 11(2):1223–1230.

Sherman, C. and Boss, P. (2007) Spousal dementia caregiving in the context of late-life remarriage. *Dementia* 6(2):245–270.

Shim, B., Barroso, J. and Davis, L.L. (2012) A comparative qualitative analysis of stories of spousal caregivers of people with dementia: Negative, ambivalent, and positive experiences. *International Journal of Nursing Studies*. doi: 10.1016/j.ijnurstu.2011.09.003

Staal, R., (2006) *What Shall We Do With Mother?: How to Manage When Your Elderly Parent Is Dependent on You*. Devon: White Ladder Press.

Walters, A., Oyebode, J. and Riley, G. (2010) The dynamics of continuity and discontinuity for women caring for a spouse with dementia. *Dementia* 9(2):169–189.

Ward, R., Vass, A., Aggarwal, N., Garfield, C. and Cybyk, B. (2005) A kiss is still a kiss? The construction of sexuality in dementia care. *Dementia* 4(1):49–72.

Watson, B., Tatangelo, G. and McCabe, M. (2019) Depression and anxiety among partner and offspring carers of people with dementia: A systematic review. *The Gerontologist* 59(5):e597–e610. doi.org/10.1093/geront/gny049

Westwood, S. (ed.) (2016) *Lesbian, Gay, Bisexual and Trans Individuals Living with Dementia: Concepts, Practice and Rights*. London and New York: Routledge and Taylor & Francis Group.

Youell, J., Callaghan, J.E.M. and Buchanan, K. (2016) "I don't know if you want to know this": Carers' understandings of intimacy in long-term relationships when one partner has dementia. *Ageing and Society* 36(5):946–967. doi: 10.1017/S0144686X15000045

5

SUPPORTING THE PERSON LIVING WITH DEMENTIA AND THEIR CARE SUPPORTER TOGETHER

We have considered the post-diagnostic support needs of the individual with dementia and also considered what may impact on partners' and family members' experiences of providing post-diagnostic support. However, it is also important to consider the needs and support of the person with the diagnosis of dementia and their care supporter together. Research has explored the wellbeing of both the person with dementia and the caregiver in relation to one another (Keady and Nolan, 2003; Robinson et al., 2005; Hellstrom et al., 2007). This kind of approach, looking at the person with dementia and the care partner, is often termed a 'dyad', that is, the recognition that the person with dementia and the care partners are interconnected and function together as well as individuals. This is not to deny that individual support and different adjustments may take place for either the person living with dementia or their care supporters. However, supporting the relationship between the person with dementia and whoever provides support to them not only creates opportunities to 'level' the playing field again and for the 'care' aspect of the relationship to not be centre stage, but it also recognises the interdependence of each person's wellbeing on the other (Keyes et al., 2018). In a study exploring spouses' experiences, Hellstrom et al. (2007) identified the efforts made by the spouses to maintain and, where possible, enhance the quality of their lives together for as long as possible. Four interlinking strategies were noted: talking things through, being appreciative and affectionate, making the best of things and keeping the peace. While this was a small study and it only explored the experiences of those in positive relationships, it does move beyond notions of burden and stress to explore the joint efforts to maintain couplehood within the caring process.

In an early review of studies focusing on the relationship between the person with dementia and the person providing care, the authors found that the voice of the person with dementia was muted in relation to the voices of those providing care (Ablitt et al., 2009). This demonstrates the need to ensure that the views and experiences of people living with dementia are given equal consideration when conducting work focusing on the relationship between dyads.

Since then research has strived to give voice to both the person with dementia and the care partner. The importance of maintaining the marital relationship has been identified as important to both the person with dementia and their partner (Clare et al., 2012) and perceptions of relationship quality are a key factor in wellbeing. Merrick et al.'s (2013) study also demonstrates the efforts couples go to both to maintain the abilities of the person with dementia and to retain their relationship. These examples clearly illustrate that the person with dementia and their spouse actively seek to work together to cope with and adjust to dementia and the impact this has for their relationship and sense of 'togetherness'. Molyneaux et al. (2011) found that couples reconstruct their relationships as they adapt to and adjust to one partner having dementia using strategies of normalising, externalising, sharing the experience and reframing the experience in light of the past. In these ways couples were able to negotiate their relationship and changes in the dynamics between them that had arisen due to dementia. In a large cohort study in the UK, Rippon et al. (2019) found that the quality of the relationship between the person with dementia and the person providing care was important to both partners, but that the self-reported views on the relationship held by the other did not impact on their perceived life satisfaction. This study is important as it provides evidence from a large-scale study about the importance of the relationship for both partners.

The interdependence between spouses and the impact this may have on who is providing care to whom is one aspect of relationships.

For example, the person with dementia may become the person providing the care, as this short account from Lesley demonstrates.

When the person who does not have dementia needs support

Lesley's story

My husband Sam was my carer, however he was diagnosed with pancreatic cancer and was very ill. I became his carer and nobody understood how hard this was for me. As I had been a nurse for 38 years the professionals thought I was coping well but nobody ever asked me, they just presumed I was coping. I wasn't, but I didn't want him to go into the hospice and he didn't want to go in either. It was really hard me watching the only man I had ever loved every day suffering severe pain. As dementia is an unseen condition and you look well, people don't see how hard it is for you to cope.

SUPPORTING THE PERSON WITH DEMENTIA AND THE CAREGIVER DYAD

As the importance of the relationship between the person living with dementia and their care supporters has been increasingly recognised, so to have approaches aimed at providing groups or interventions designed to support the person with dementia and their care partners together.

Australian research has demonstrated that the person living with dementia and their partner (the dyad) undergo a process of loss and adjustment as a couple and that fear of how others will react impacts on how they self-manage dementia (Stockwell-Smith et al., 2019). They argue that interventions are needed to prevent the breakdown of the relationship and to reduce stress within the relationship. In this way people may be supported to successfully self-manage dementia within the relationship.

An example of an approach to support couples with dementia (Hill et al., 2018) is a programme of sessions focusing on the couple and their relationship that had the explicit aim of reinforcing each couple's relationship and to help the couple to navigate and work together to develop their own strategies to cope with dementia. This initiative was positively evaluated by all participants and demonstrates the value of focusing on the couple, rather than just the person with dementia or the care supporter. The authors argue that this kind of approach has the potential to enable couples to self-manage and navigate the relational challenges that accompany the diagnosis and symptoms of dementia.

Music is a particularly powerful way for people to connect to one another. Another example of a group designed for the person living with dementia and their partners are singing groups (Camic et al., 2013) where both partners were able to actively participate and enjoy an 'in-the-moment' experience with one another (Unadkat et al., 2017). Being able to participate in leisure opportunities together has been found to be a key source of reported satisfaction for both the person living with dementia and the care partner (Innes et al., 2016), where as a family/couple individuals can go out and visit places of interest, whether these are castles, beaches, parks or other local attractions close to where they live. Accessing heritage groups as a dyad, where both the person with dementia and the care partner have attended sessions where they learn and participate in sensory activities as a partnership have also been reported as beneficial (Scholar et al., 2019). Viewing and making art together in groups designed for dyads have also been perceived positively by the person with dementia and their care partner (Camic et al., 2014).

Lesley's reflections on the different activities she attended with her late husband demonstrate how these benefitted her as an individual and her relationship.

The benefits of the groups attended by Lesley and her late husband, Sam

To start with I went to groups with my husband, Sam. We made friends in these groups and I kept going on my own after he died. Being part of the dementia associates at Salford University has given me a place to go and keep my brain stimulated. As part of the university I have been part of the new nursing curriculum. I speak to the first- and second-year students about what it is like living with dementia, from how it first affected me, to how I got my diagnosis, losing my car, job and independence, to how I live my life today. I have also been a speaker at other conferences at the university. I must say these are things I would never have thought about doing before I had dementia and Sam encouraged me to take part in everything.

I have also been asked to speak to students at Manchester University. This makes me feel that, even though I have dementia, I can still give to the nursing profession that was a large part of my life. I am asked regularly to speak to groups of district nurses in the Salford area where I worked. I think often how much more impact it would have had on me if when I was working somebody would have come and explained how hard it was to live with dementia but how much easier it is if people in general knew and could help you.

I am part of Greater Manchester Dementia United Implementation Operations group as a person living with dementia. This is a large project which covers everything that can make it easier to live well, such as transport, lived experience, delirium and end of life, to name a few. It doesn't matter where in Greater Manchester you live; if you have dementia then you will get the same treatment, and if you move you will still carry on with the same journey. This is important as people with dementia don't like change of any kind. I also go to Open Doors dementia café and post-diagnostic group. We have also been involved in research looking at our neighbourhood and how it's changed from when we were children. This is easy, as my long-term memory at the moment is very good. Meeting with anybody just improves my wellbeing.

Much of the literature focuses on spouse/partner relationships and activities designed to support both the person with dementia and their care partner. However, it is not just spouse/partner relationships that can be maintained by initiatives designed for both the care partner and the person living with dementia. At the University of Salford we have various groups designed for both the person with dementia and their care supporters, whether they are spouses or another family member. Gail provides an account here of the importance of attending groups with her father and the benefit to their relationship.

The importance of the groups Gail attends with her father, Ron

Dad's dementia has been on a plateau since 2015, meaning that he still has capacity. However, one symptom of his condition is separation anxiety, and it can be extreme. Due to this dad and I are joined at the hip, and finding groups and dementia cafés that suited both our needs proved very difficult at the beginning of our journey. Most were only for the person living with dementia, and carers' groups were not specific to dementia. I also found that many of the groups for dad were not stimulating enough for him, and to be honest, could not offer him what he needed, as he is visually impaired and in a wheelchair. There were lots of exercise groups, dance groups, creative arts and singing, but these were not appropriate and the singing groups were too noisy and the music wasn't of dad's preferred genre.

That was until I visited the Institute for Dementia at Salford University. It was like a breath of fresh air; the staff were friendly and those using the institute were warm and welcoming. Dad wasn't with me on this first visit, but I knew that I had found the perfect place where we could both come and enjoy the activities and the company. The institute provides creative arts that I enjoy, gardening and use of outdoor space which we both like, and music which is also our passion. We are associates now, which means that we also engage with researchers and academics from across the dementia arena, using our experiences to affect change and drive forward reform.

Dad looks forward to his visits to the institute; you could say that it is the highlight of his week. It not only provides stimulus, but he is treated with dignity and respect, and his dementia isn't seen. Dad is seen for who he is and that is very important. He says that he always feels wanted whilst with all the participants and staff. He knows that his opinions are valued and if he has a good time, this feeling lasts longer than just the time spent at the institute. Our favourite days are those where we make music or have musicians coming in to play to the group. Dad was a musician – drums and percussion, so he appreciates the value of music and the therapeutic properties it holds.

Having access to groups is imperative for our overall health and wellbeing. On a personal level, I can be feeling down, but once at the institute I feel happy and uplifted. Seeing people enjoying themselves in an environment which is safe, warm and inviting is endearing.

In this chapter of the book we have highlighted the increasing recognition of the importance of the relationship between the person with the diagnosis of dementia and their care supporters. Groups and initiatives designed to support the person with dementia and their spouse/partner have evolved in the last decade. Less evidence exists about the benefits on relationships between the person with dementia and non-spouse/partner carers and the impact groups may have on those relationships and feelings of wellbeing. It is important to recognise that sometimes people living with dementia will want to be with a care partner/supporter and at other times they may not. Also, those providing care may enjoy doing activities with the person with dementia but may also benefit from time away from the care supporter role. What is important is that the needs of both the person with dementia and the care supporters are recognised and that appropriate services and groups are available to meet individual and joint support needs. These may vary over the dementia journey as symptoms of dementia progress and change over time and care partners' coping mechanisms and their own health and support needs may evolve. This section of the book has looked at post-diagnostic support from the perspective of the person living with dementia, the care partners and the person with dementia and care partners together. In the next section of the book we will explore how, as the dementia journey progresses, there may be transitions in the post-diagnostic support that people may require (chapter 6) and also consider what is required if the person living with dementia needs end of life care (chapter 7).

REFERENCES

Ablitt, A., Jones, G. and Muersc, J. (2009) Living with dementia: A systematic review of the influence of relationship factors. *Aging & Mental Health* 13(4):497–511.

Camic, P.M., Tischler, V. and Pearman, C.H. (2014) Viewing and making art together: A multi-session art-gallery-based intervention for people with dementia and their carers. *Aging & Mental Health* 18(2):161–168.

Camic, P.M., Williams, C.M. and Meeten, F. (2013) Does a "Singing together group" improve the quality of life of people with a dementia and their carers? A pilot evaluation study. *Dementia* 12:157–176. doi: 10.1177/1471301211422761

Clare, L., Nelis, S., Whitaker, C.J., Martyr, A., Markova, I.S., Roth, I., Woods, R.T. and Morris, R.G. (2012) Marital relationship quality in early-stage dementia: Perspectives from people with dementia and their spouses. *Alzheimer Disease & Associated Disorders* 26(2):148–158.

Hellstrom, I., Nolan, M. and Lundh, U. (2007) Sustaining "couplehood": Spouses' strategies for living positively with dementia. *Dementia* 6(3):383–409.

Hill, H., Yeates, S. and Donovan, J. (2018) You, me, us: Creating connection: Report on a program to support and empower couples to navigate the challenges of dementia (innovative practice). *Dementia*. doi: 10.1177/1471301218786592

Innes, A., Page, S.J. and Cutler, C. (2016) Barriers to leisure participation for people with dementia and their carers: An exploratory analysis of carer and people with dementias experiences. *Dementia* 15(6):1643–1665. doi: 10.1177/1471301215570346

Keady, J. and Nolan, M. (2003) The dynamics of dementia: Working together, working separately or working alone? In Nolan, M., Lundh, U., Grant, G. and Keady, J. (Eds.), *Partnerships in Family Care*. Maidenhead: Open University Press.

Keyes, S.E., Clarke, C.L. and Gibb, C.E. (2018) Living with dementia, interdependence and citizenship: Narratives of everyday decision-making. *Disability and Society* 34(2):296–319. https://doi.org/10.1080/09687599.2018.1528970

Lipinska, D. (2017) *Dementia, Sex and Wellbeing: A Person-Centred Guide for People with Dementia, Their Partners, Caregivers and Professionals*. London: Jessica Kingsley.

McCabe, L., Robertson, J. and Kelly, F. (2018) Scaffolding and working together: A qualitative exploration of strategies for everyday life with dementia. *Age and Ageing* 47(2):303–310. doi.org/10.1093/ageing/afx186

Merrick, K., Camic, P.M. and O'Shaughnessy, M. (2013) Couples constructing their experiences of dementia: A relational perspective. *Dementia*. doi:10.1177/1471301213513029

Molyneaux, V.J., Butchard, S., Simpson, S. and Murray, C. (2011) The co-construction of couplehood in dementia. *Dementia* 11(4):483–502.

Rippon, I., Quinn, C., Martyr, A., Morris, R., Nelis, S.M., Jones, I.R., Victor, C.R. and Linda Clare on behalf of the IDEAL programme (2019) The impact of relationship quality on life satisfaction and well-being in dementia caregiving dyads: Findings from the IDEAL study. *Aging & Mental Health*. doi: 10.1080/13607863.2019.1617238

Robinson, L., Clare, L. and Evans, K. (2005) Making sense of dementia and adjusting to loss: Psychological reactions to a diagnosis of dementia in couples. *Aging & Mental Health* 9(4):337–347.

Scholar, H., Innes, A., Haragalova, J. and Sharma, S. (2019) "Unlocking the door to being there": The contribution of creative facilitators in supporting people living with dementia to engage with heritage settings. *Dementia*. https://doi.org/10.1177/1471301219871388

Stockwell-Smith, G., Moyle, W. and Kellett, U. (2019) The impact of early-stage dementia on community-dwelling care recipient/carer dyads' capacity to self-manage. *Journal of Clinical Nursing* 28(3):629–640.

Unadkat, S., Camic, P. and Vella-Burrows, T. (2017) Understanding the experience of group singing for couples where one partner has a diagnosis of dementia. *Gerontologist* 57(3):469–478. doi: 10.1093/geront/gnv698

SECTION 3
CARE TRANSITIONS

The journey of dementia is one that can progress to the point where individuals with the diagnosis and their families require additional support to the initial post-diagnostic support that they accessed. This can be due to their needs developing over time and support changes required to maintain their participation in social life and promote and maintain their wellbeing. In this section of the book we will consider the transitions that may happen over time as the person with dementia requires increased or different support as well as the various roles family care supporters may take on over time (chapter 6). We will also consider the move from living at home in the community to a care home or admission to hospital. In chapter 7 we will specifically consider end of life care.

6

CARE NEED TRANSITIONS IN THE JOURNEY WITH DEMENTIA

Changes over time, or specific transition points, from needing formal day care provision to respite care to long-term care, like a care home placement, can be difficult for the person living with dementia and their family members, and many do not receive the support and information they need for a smooth transition. The supports required can vary, from respite support for the family members providing ongoing care and support to the person living with dementia who remains at home, to requiring additional day care and accessing other services in the community, such as speech therapy, occupational therapy and other community-based services. Sometimes a crisis situation has been the precursor to, or trigger, for increased care and support – for example if the family member or the person living with dementia becomes ill. Or an incident occurs such as the person with dementia getting lost or no longer being able to carry out activities of daily living such as cooking, shopping and personal care. Or, both the person with dementia and their family supporters become concerned with safety in the home, for example forgetting to turn off the gas when cooking, or when outside, for example, being unable to find their way home or to a point of safety. Adapting to the need for increased support can be a difficult transition for all concerned. There may also be an increase in use of GP and hospital visits due to either the symptoms of dementia or concurrent conditions.

It may also be necessary to review the care needs and where these can best be met, and this may lead up to a decision for the person with dementia to move into a long-term care facility, such as housing with extra care or a care home. Moving from home to a care home can be a traumatic time for the person living with dementia and for family members. There are different reasons for this and there can also be different outcomes. There may be feelings of grief, guilt, relief and sorrow for everyone concerned.

EMOTIONAL FEELINGS: LOSS, GUILT AND AN ONGOING BEREAVEMENT PROCESS

Feelings of guilt and loss can be very strong not just when either the person with dementia or the care supporter dies but when the person requires different support. Bereavement can become an ongoing process (Adams and Sanders, 2004) where the family member can grieve for the loss or change in a relationship and feel guilty for no longer having the ability to provide care at home (Blandin and Pepin, 2018). The recognition of an ongoing grief or bereavement process has been recognised and some attempts have begun to try and provide support (MacCourt et al., 2017; Owen and Dening, 2018) for what has been called 'anticipatory grief' (Walker et al., 1997), that is, grief that occurs before the physical death of the person living with dementia. Although anticipatory grief has been found to be most acute as the person nears end of life, it has also been found to be present as care needs and support needs develop (Cheung et al., 2018).

The person with dementia can also feel guilt at placing demands on their family members and friends and be concerned about being a burden on others. This is often one of the reasons that people living with dementia seek to create advance care plans and 'get their house in order' to reduce the burden on their families (Dickinson et al., 2013). In addition, the care partner of the person living with dementia may become ill and die and the person with dementia can experience bereavement and loss that can be difficult to process due to memory recall.

TRANSITION POINT: INCREASED CARE AND SUPPORT NEEDS

Sometimes it may be the person with dementia who develops increased care and support needs, either because of the progress of their dementia, or due to other conditions and complex co-morbidities resulting in changes to the way they can manage at home independently with the support of family members and friends. Or it may be that the person providing the support and care experiences health problems or simply begins to find the ongoing pressures of providing care too much to continue without some support and care for their needs as individuals. Whatever the reason, reaching out and asking for more support and help can be difficult, and even when explorations are made as to what other support might be available the experience can be difficult if services and groups that might be available locally do not match the requirements as perceived by the person with dementia and the care supporters.

Gail's story

As you journey through dementia you realise that as a carer you can't do everything yourself. As a fiercely independent person I found it hard to ask for help, but knew that if I didn't I could quite easily end up at a crisis point, which would have been detrimental for my parents as well as for me.

I had already experienced a lot, such as mum's paranoia, hallucinations and mood swings, all of which occurred at the earlier stages of her dementia, and which were controlled with medication and love. But as the disease progressed mum's physical abilities started to be affected, such as her ability to walk and swallow. I knew that to be able to help her I needed to look at professional interventions such as physiotherapy, speech and language therapy and the GP.

With dad, his transitions are very different to those mum went through. So, as a carer I felt that I was prepared; however, dad has multiple morbidities which affect his overall general health. Due to these conditions dad has had several admissions into hospital and has regular interventions from the district nurses and the GP.

Gerry, Gail's mum's, story

Thankfully as mum's dementia progressed, she never tried to walk out of the house on her own, so there was never an occasion to call the police. As it happened her mobility was greatly affected due to the dementia. Her stance became stooped and she would shuffle rather than walk. We also had a number of occasions where she would drop to her knees so I would have to gently lower her to the floor. This was to stop her falling but made it difficult to stand again. I spoke with the GP, district nurse and CPN about this, and a physiotherapist was assigned to us. I also arranged for a falls pendant through the council's care-on-call team. This meant that if she was on the floor, I could contact them, and they used a device called a *mangar* – an inflatable cushion. The mangar was placed under mum then inflated so that she was raised off the floor, enabling the team to lift her onto the chair or bed.

David the physiotherapist was brilliant; he encouraged mum to walk with a walking aid, and I think he only had success because she flirted with him, as she had a thing for dark-haired, bearded men! He also tried to encourage mum to walk down the stairs, but this was to no avail as she became too frightened of the stairs, believing that they were a sheer drop.

The next intervention came from the speech and language thera-pist, as mum started to have problems with her swallowing. Thank-fully she wasn't aspirating, but she was finding it difficult to eat. There were two factors behind this – the dementia and the cancer she had. The therapist taught me ways of feeding mum – using a small spoon and giving her a soft diet – and how to encourage her to swallow by gently stroking her throat. The GP also advised to just give her what she wanted, so if she was struggling with normal food then give her ice cream or a dessert that she enjoyed. As long as she was taking in food, the professionals were not bothered what it was. The ethos was that it was quality of life at this point.

Mum was not admitted into hospital at any stage of her illness. This was due to the advance care plan, which stated that all treat-ments or interventions should take place in the community. Towards the end of mum's life, the GP and the district nurses visited more frequently – this was to oversee pain management and to ensure that she was comfortable. The hospice-at-home team also visited more, so dad and I could have some respite in preparation of what lay ahead.

Mum had been living with her dementia for many years before her cancer diagnosis. Due to her dementia she was fearful of transport, and she absolutely dreaded the thought of having to attend hospital.

We first knew that something was wrong when her right leg began to swell to more than double its size. The GP at the time was a trainee, but he understood dementia, and more importantly he began to understand mum. He told me that mum required a scan, but not to worry as he had a plan to get us to the hospital.

When the day arrived for the trip to outpatients, the GP had arranged for a transport ambulance to come for us. He had already spoken to the staff and explained our situation. The staff were brilliant. They came into the house with beaming smiles and greeted mum with warmth and compassion. They said that they had a bus outside ready to take her away for the day. They linked arms with mum down the path and to the 'bus', helped her to step in and made sure her seat belt was fastened. I went too, and they carried on the ruse all the way to the hospital. Fortunately, the hospital's entrance doesn't resemble anything like a hospital or clinic. It has gardens, a water feature and shops in the main concourse. All of this helped to keep mum calm, and she believed up to this point that she was somewhere nice for the day.

This made all the difference, because mum was not anxious, and as we waited in the waiting room, the staff again made sure that mum felt as if she was somewhere other than a hospital. They made her cups of tea and even brought her a cupcake. One of the reception staff came and sat beside her, asking about her toy dog that we had to bring along for the ride! When we were called for the scan, that's when things took a downturn, as she was taken into a small examination room. There were two nurses, who, though kind, really didn't understand dementia. They lacked the patience and empathy required to communicate effectively with mum, so she became distressed. Thankfully the scan didn't take very long, and we were taken back to the waiting room.

The receptionist saw that mum was distressed, so came over and held her hand. She asked if she would like a cup of tea, and further went on to talk about mum's 'dog'. The consultant then came in to see me, so the receptionist said that she would stay with mum, so I could chat with the doctor. That's when I was told that she had cancer, but due to the severity of her dementia, only palliative treatment would be given. The journey home was upsetting for me, as I knew that I had to break the news to my dad, but the ambulance staff were great again with mum. They chatted about all sorts of things with her.

It is the small kind gestures and understanding of the situation that go a long way. I will not forget the kindness of these individuals, as it was their compassion that got me as a carer through the day.

Transitions in the journey with dementia: Gail's dad

Dad's dementia has been on a plateau since his diagnosis in 2015. He still has mental capacity and can still make decisions, which meant that he fully participated in developing his advance care plan. It states that where applicable all treatment is to take place in the community unless it is felt that a hospital admission would have a positive outcome. With this in mind dad was placed on the Gold Standard Framework, which means that all NHS professionals involved in dad's care are aware that he has multiple morbidities as well as dementia. It also means that the GP has a greater input into dad's care and we have district nurse intervention.

Dad has been a 'frequent flyer' over the past three years at our local hospital. He was admitted five times for sepsis and has had several bouts of pneumonia. Following on from his last stay in hospital he also acquired three separate hospital infections due to his compromised immune system. Hospital admissions bear their own risks for dad, hence the ACP. We have also found that hospitals are not the right environment for a person with dementia. They are confusing places, full of noise and light, causing stimulus overload. There is too much stimulus and the risk for dad to acquire a delirium is heightened.

Dad has also had to use the services of the speech and language therapy team due to aspiration. He has a delayed swallow, which means that some liquid finds its way to his lungs. To prevent this from happening, dad now has to have thickened fluids, though his diet is normal. Since being in hospital for nine weeks, dad also lost his mobility. It was poor before going into hospital, but now we have to live downstairs in our home, and we also have to use a standing aid, wheelchair and rise and fall bed. Due to this dad has to be regularly assessed by occupational therapists and the district nurses.

Thankfully we can still enjoy days out and attending the numerous clubs and societies we belong to. For how long, that's anyone's guess, but as long as dad wants to, we will. I know that due to his various health issues there is a chance of a rapid decline, and when that time comes, I am aware that the professional bodies will have to step up and offer me more assistance. But until then it's business as usual!

Lesley's story

When I was first diagnosed with dementia, I knew I would be alright as I was in the early stages of dementia, however, I now have to think what I need to do and what help I need as time goes on.

I have always said that I don't want to go into any residential or nursing home. So how do I prevent this? I have told my son and daughter my wishes. They have also been written down when I wrote my power of attorney. I wrote that I don't want resuscitating if at any time from diagnosis I have a cardiac arrest; also I don't want artificial feeding. This does not mean I want to be denied fluids; I am happy to have intravenous fluids as a temporary measure if I should get a sepsis or other infection. It would be cruel for any person to be denied fluids as it would be a slow, long, drawn-out death.

Whilst I am able, I have moved nearer to my daughter so if she needs to help me more than at present it won't be as stressful for her, as I don't want to be a burden. I wouldn't mind going to day care as long as I am able to move about. I love walking and to be restrained would cause me to get stressed and angry. I have heard carers saying 'she/he is wandering' when all they are doing is walking round. I find it hard to sleep and living on my own, I spend a large part of the night walking round the house. I am certainly not wandering, I'm walking.

There are a lot of devices available today that can help people with dementia to carry on living independently. I would rather use these than go into a residential home. I already have problems with the cooking, shopping and personal care but when my daughter isn't able to help, I pay another carer to help me with these activities of daily living. Cooking is the most dangerous for me as I have set the grill on fire after forgetting I had put it on, not realising until I saw the smoke coming out of the back door, so now I don't use the cooker at all.

I feel it's hard for me because what I want might not be what I get as I get older, as my children's health might also deteriorate, so looking after me might not be an option.

Another thing I worry about is if I have another illness and it is just put down to a deterioration of the dementia when it is a deterioration of another health condition I have, that can be cured. This could be because I am not able to speak for myself.

When does the person with dementia become the carer? This happened to me a few years ago. My husband, Sam, became my carer when I was diagnosed and did the shopping and cooking, but he took ill with pancreatic cancer and I became his carer. We really struggled, but I didn't want him to go into a hospice; he didn't either, but was worried I couldn't cope. I thought we would get more help from the caring services, but I was wrong. For three months we struggled through until he died. I am still angry to this day that the services let us down. However, I did have help from friends and extended family, or I don't think I could have looked after Sam at home.

I think the reason help wasn't forthcoming was because I was a nurse before I was diagnosed with dementia. They all thought I was able to care for Sam but they forgot that I was living with dementia and my brain wasn't functioning as it should.

Planning for the future

When we attended the post-diagnostic support group part of it was about making a will and power of attorney. At the time we thought it was a bit premature to do this. However, I can honestly say this was one of the best things we did, as both my husband and I made wills and set up power of attorney. In the end it wasn't for me that we had to use it, but for my husband, who was given three months to live when diagnosed with pancreatic cancer. My daughter and son took over and when he died it was so easy for all the finances to be sorted quickly, which supported me as there was no stress.

Having also made a power of attorney for health I have written down all that I want while I have the capacity to do this, such as not being resuscitated if I should collapse with a heart attack and not being tube fed if I can't feed myself. This has taken the responsibility of making the decision from my children, so they don't have to decide what to do when they are in a distressed state.

I have also stated that I don't ever want to go into a care or nursing home. That I want to stay in my own home where I know where everything is and where I feel safe. However, I do know this might not be how it works out, as people in authority such as hospital doctors might be able to overturn my wishes if the new liberty protection safeguards get through Parliament.

Recently I returned to the local memory service for my six-month check up with my daughter, who is now my carer. During this appointment she opened up for the first time in three years since she took over the care from her dad and spoke of how looking after me was causing her concern and that she felt she wasn't coping well. After I went to live with her, I think she realised that caring for me is more of a struggle than she thought it would be. She has now asked for help. I try my best but the moods that I have change from day to day as I try to remember more than one thing. This has made me think – what is life going to be like for her, and for me when I am not able to help a little? I have always said I don't want to move into a care home and this is still how I feel. However, my daughter needs a life as much as I do and although I have always stated what I want, as things change I am thinking now this won't be how it ends up.

These personal accounts demonstrate the different care and support needs that may evolve over time and the responses by the person living with dementia and family members to these changes. Our examples are from people with strong family relationships. If family relationships are already strained or fractured in any way or become strained due to the demands of caregiving (O'Reilly and Shatz, 2019), this can lead to considerable stress for both the person living with dementia and for family members (Tatangelo et al., 2018). The dynamics between family members and the person with dementia are important and will impact on the way families choose to work together to provide support and care (Innes et al., 2011). Therefore, the availability of support and care away from the home can be critical for the wellbeing of everyone concerned.

TRANSITION POINT: NEEDING TO GO INTO HOSPITAL OR A CARE HOME

With an ageing population, increasing incidence of dementia and government policy aimed at keeping people living in their own homes for longer (DoH, 2009; Alzheimer Disease International, 2016), it is perhaps inevitable that people with dementia (particularly older, frailer people) will at some stage need to be admitted to hospital for a short time. Transitions are not stages but periods of movement from one state or place to another, and the move to a hospital setting, for example when an injury or accident has taken place, can be traumatic. We will consider practical and emotional issues that may accompany the transition to hospital, a time that is likely to be traumatic for family members and the person living with dementia.

Reasons for hospital admission

The majority of older people with dementia live in the community and like other older people living in the community, are likely to access hospital care, particularly in-patient, out-patient and accident and emergency services as a result of a decline or crisis in acute and/or chronic health conditions (Alzheimer's Society, 2009). The Alzheimer's Society (2009) estimates that people with dementia over the age of 65 use one-quarter of hospital beds at any one time. It is clear from this that hospital staff are likely to encounter a patient who has dementia, and often a distressed family member, in most areas of a hospital. People living with dementia are one of the highest users of hospitals (Sampson et al., 2009) and the costs associated with providing care for people living with dementia in hospital are three times higher than for people who do not have dementia (Briggs et al., 2015).

Common reasons for admission to hospital are falls, infection or acute medical or surgical problems; another reason is delirium. The UK National Institute of Clinical Excellence (NICE) states that:

> Delirium (sometimes called 'acute confusional state') is a common clinical syndrome characterised by disturbed consciousness, cognitive function or perception, which has an acute onset and fluctuating course. It usually develops over 1–2 days. It is a serious condition that is associated with poor outcomes. However, it can be prevented and treated if dealt with urgently.

Causes of delirium include infection, constipation, dehydration, injury, disease, medications, alcohol or poisons. The NICE guideline (2019) has identified people with dementia as at risk of delirium and estimates that 10 to 30 percent of people in hospital have this. Delirium is typified by a rapid change in cognition and is characterised by hallucination, sleep disturbance, clouding of consciousness and misinterpretation of events. Differentiating between dementia and delirium is crucial, as is identifying delirium in someone with dementia, because the causes of delirium can be treated once identified.

Consequences of hospital admission

The particular needs of people with dementia are often unrecognised and poorly understood by health care staff working in general medical settings, such as general hospital wards, who have had little training in this area (Scerri et al., 2017; Moyle et al., 2011). Emergency departments are often difficult places for people living with dementia, with recent research reporting that they are under-triaged and left waiting and worrying about what is wrong; that there is time pressure with lack of attention to basic needs; and, that relationships and interactions with staff lead people to feel ignored, forgotten and unimportant (Parke et al., 2013). There is little work exploring how people living with dementia and their families perceive hospital stays but the studies that have explored this have found that their perceptions are that quality of care is poor (Featherstone et al., 2019; Scerri et al., 2018; Porock et al., 2015). Critiques of hospital care for older people have found that a lack of appropriately trained staff and endemic ageism lead to a loss of dignity, reduced autonomy and neglect (Scerri et al., 2018). Innes et al. (2016) found that hospital staff in wards with older people with dementia had negative perceptions of people living with dementia, and that their perceptions of the care being offered were quite different to the care experience observed. Moyle et al.'s (2011) Australian research found that staff untrained in dementia were trying to promote safety (or avert risk) at the expense of patient wellbeing and dignity. This finding was echoed in Maltese research (Scerri et al., 2018) where staff felt preventing risk was more important than promoting choice.

People with dementia use hospitals in the highest numbers, and they generally experience worse outcomes following an episode of acute hospital care than those without dementia (Sampson et al., 2009; Briggs et al., 2015; Dewing and Dijk, 2016), with higher rates of delirium and death (Sampson et al., 2013), longer stays and more dehydration and malnutrition (Dewing and Dijk, 2016). The Alzheimer's Society (2009) study looking at hospital care found that:

- Ninety-seven percent of nursing staff and nurse managers reported that they always or sometimes care for someone with dementia.
- Seventy-seven percent of nurse managers and nursing staff said that antipsychotic drugs were used always or sometimes to treat people with dementia in the hospital environment. Of those nurse managers and nursing staff who said that antipsychotics were used, up to a quarter thought that they were not appropriately prescribed to people with dementia.

- Eighty-six percent of nurse managers felt that people with dementia either always or sometimes have a longer stay in hospital than people without dementia admitted with the same medical condition.

The report concluded that the longer people with dementia are in hospital, the worse the effect on the symptoms of dementia and physical health; discharge to a care home becomes more likely and antipsychotic drugs are more likely to be used. Thus, additional financial pressure is placed on hospitals by people with dementia staying in hospital longer than expected or required.

Family member experiences

In the foreword to the Alzheimer's Society (2009, vii) report on caring for people with dementia in acute hospital wards, Angela Rippon says:

> Seeing my mother in hospital was one of the hardest times in my life. I remember being struck with a desperate sorrow watching how vulnerable and helpless she was in an unfamiliar environment. Her battle was not just with the emphysema and bronchitis: it was with the strange environment, the people she didn't know and the intrusive medication she couldn't understand. There were frightening and scary moments. She was so dependent on those who were caring for her. But she was incredibly brave; that's my mother.

This is a moving account of the distress carers can face when their family member is admitted to the unfamiliar environment of an accident and emergency department or a hospital ward. In their report, the Alzheimer's Society (2009) found that:

- Forty-seven percent of carer respondents said that being in hospital had a significant negative effect on the general physical health of the person with dementia, which wasn't a direct result of the medical condition.
- Seventy-seven percent of carer respondents were dissatisfied with the overall quality of dementia care provided.
- Fifty-four percent of carer respondents said that being in hospital had a significant negative effect on the symptoms of dementia, such as becoming more confused and less independent.

- Forty-nine percent of carer respondents said that the hospital stay was overall longer than they expected it to be.
- Over a third of people with dementia who go into hospital from living in their own homes are discharged to a care home setting.

Partly in response to concerns about hospital admissions and stay experiences, health care policy has evolved in recognition of the need to improve care in hospitals on a general ward and to move care away from costly acute settings into the community. The first English National Dementia Strategy (Department of Health, 2009) had two objectives focusing on hospital admissions. Objective 8 outlined the need to improve the quality of care for people with dementia in general hospitals by identifying leadership for dementia, defining the care pathway for dementia and commissioning specialist liaison older people's mental health teams to work in general hospitals. Objective 9 outlined the need for improved intermediate care for people with dementia to avoid initial unnecessary hospitalisation and to enable a pathway out of hospital. Kelley et al.'s (2019) recent study exploring family involvement in hospital care for people living with dementia found that when involved, there were positive outcomes for the person living with dementia and for the family members. However, this involvement was not routine and was not supported by hospital staff. Research demonstrates that involving families while the person is in hospital can help the person living with dementia to stay connected and can enhance communication and knowledge sharing with hospital staff (Kelley et al., 2019; Porock et al., 2015). Doing so enables a continuation of the support most people living with dementia receive in the community while in hospital. Given that the focus on supporting people at home in the community is common internationally (Alzheimer Disease International, 2016), drawing on the skills and expertise of families and friends is important to facilitate when there is a need for hospital admissions. Therefore it is important that hospitals continue to work to improve the care they offer to people living with dementia and their families. Encouraging the involvement of families and drawing on their extensive knowledge of the person with dementia may be one way to bring about improvements in the experiences in hospitals of people living with dementia and their families.

Transition to a care home

The decision to move a relative into a care home can be stressful and carers may need support. Canadian research found that this decision was one of the most difficult for families to make (Caron et al., 2006). Similarly in Chinese research (Chang et al., 2011), this was a decision that led to conflict amongst families as they debated the best course of action and decided that care at home was no longer viable. A review of 15 studies exploring the needs of family members during this time (Afram et al., 2015) concluded that family members need support handling the emotions that arise through such decisions, for example feelings of grief or shame, a need for more knowledge or information about care home processes and a need for more support (e.g. counselling) as they adjust to a different role in the support of the person living with dementia. The decision to place a person living with dementia in a care home can often be taken out of their hands in a crisis situation such as deteriorating health resulting in a hospital admission that then leads to a care home admission, or the sudden illness or death of the primary family member providing support and care. Regardless of the circumstances this is often a period that family members find very difficult, even if the person with dementia requires the 24-hour help of care professionals that cannot easily be provided in the person's own home.

Cho et al. (2009) found caregiving stress, carer wellbeing, gender and the carer's relationship with the person with dementia were all factors in the decision to place a relative into long-term care. Cho et al. (2009) looked specifically at the use of day care and the relationship between the carer and the person with dementia. They found that wives using day care were more likely to place their husband into residential care than a daughter caring for a parent who attended day care, but other factors such as role overload were also influential.

Historically, most of the research on decision making and care home admissions focuses on the views and experiences of family members, and have found overall that family members find proxy decision-making on behalf of the person living with dementia about care home placement both distressing and challenging, particularly when they know this is not what the person living with dementia would like (Lord et al., 2015). The views of people living with dementia about moving into a care home have been less well researched. One notable recent example looked at the views of both the person with dementia and the family members around the time the decision was being made (Lord et al., 2015). Lord et al. (2016) found that many of their participants living with dementia felt that the decision was being made for them and resented this. Others understood the family members' concerns and felt they had been included in the discussions; even if they would rather stay in their own homes, they had an understanding of the reasons for the decisions (e.g. safety, health issues). There seems to be few studies that have looked at the views of people living with dementia about moving into a care home, although research exploring experiences when already in care homes has demonstrated that the decision to enter the care home was not perceived to be that of the person living with dementia (e.g. Innes et al., 2011).

While relatives are concerned to find a suitable care home, they can often be faced with a lack of information and guidance for making such an important decision. Or, they find a home they like but there are no available spots. The need to have somewhere for the person living with dementia to go, for example so they can move out of hospital, can put pressure on families to choose a home based on availability rather than what they would really like.

Useful resource about experiences of moving into a care home

SCIE has a range of videos documenting family experiences of deciding to place the person living with dementia into a care home:

SCIE (2010) Working with Lesbian, Gay, Bisexual and Transgendered People – Older People and Residential Care: Roger's Story www.scie.org.uk/socialcaretv/video-player.asp?guid=cacaae 12-7375-429a-9d9a-1d28e29e65bd

SCIE (2009) Living in a Care Home: A Positive Outcome for a Person with Dementia www.scie.org.uk/socialcaretv/video-player.asp?guid=38fc468e-b6e0-4edf-b20d-979d83822f14

What happens to family members' caring role(s) when the person living with dementia is no longer at home?

The importance of involving families in care homes has been recognised for over a decade now (Woods et al., 2008). Until then, research into carers' experiences after their relative is admitted into continuing care was relatively sparse. In their review of research exploring the experiences of family members after the person living with dementia has moved to a care home, Graneheim et al. (2014) found that relinquishing the caregiving role has been reported as difficult. Many family members report finding placement into long-term care a devastating experience, often because there has been little if any forward planning and because admission into care is often in response to a crisis. Carers often claim that the admission of their relative into long-term care was an ambivalent experience with any relief they felt being tempered with feelings of guilt or failure (Rosen et al., 2019). In a review exploring the impact on quality of life on family members following the person living with dementia's placement in a nursing home Moon et al. (2017) found that for some quality of life improved as they were now able to look after themselves and experienced less stress and strain, for others however quality of life declined as the feelings of guilt and loss of their role was very difficult to navigate.

Early seminal work in this area found that:

*   Carers are both central, yet marginalised – 'your husband but my resident'.
*   Carers feel relief yet experience guilt, anger, despair and resentment.
*   Carers give information yet feel they have information withheld from them.
*   Carers need to question yet are frightened to.
*   Carers recognise staff knowledge but also have their own knowledge to pass on.

(Nay, 1996)

A subsequent review of research exploring the relationships between staff in care settings and family members found that it was important to develop initiatives to:

1   Improve staff-family perceptions of one another.
2   Reduce organisational barriers to family involvement.

3   Promote measures to improve communication between staff and family members.
4   Encourage staff to work towards ensuring that family members are present as equals in the care support role of individuals living with dementia.
5   Promote the uniqueness of each individual with dementia at all times.

(Haesler et al., 2007)

However, achieving this in practice is challenging, as the reports of the continued nature of these issues demonstrate. Care home placements are a difficult time for family members and support may be required to enable this to be navigated successfully.

There is no reason to surmise that following placement in long-term care, caregiving ceases or that the carer ceases to have a role. Overall, long-term care placement should be considered not as an end to caring, but another transition point on the continuum of care. Many carers may need active encouragement and guidance from professionals to facilitate their continued and meaningful involvement. This may necessitate a change in mindset from staff and adjustments to policies and practice to encourage true partnerships and full acknowledgement of family members' potential contribution.

Long-term care and views of people living with dementia

It is not only family members who find the move to long-term care difficult. The person with dementia might also experience feelings of loss and bereavement or difficulties associated with finding themselves in a communal living environment. Research about the views and experiences of people with dementia after the move into a care setting is relatively sparse. However, it is evident that the move into a care home or other long-term care setting is not an easy one. For example, in a study carried out in a psycho-geriatric unit with six people with moderate to advanced dementia that asked the residents about their views of living there, Edvardsson and Nordvall (2008) found that:

- Participants felt lost – not knowing where they were and why they were there.
- They felt insecure, ill at ease and personally threatened due to invasion of their space by others with dementia.
- They experienced boredom and felt devalued by care staff.

The transition from home to long-term care as a difficult time, no matter how far along the dementia is deemed to be.

The lives of people with dementia will also change in the new environment, perhaps due to new routines and the new environment, both physical and social. In a study in Norway care home residents felt homesick and that their freedom was restricted; they also felt that they were not seen or heard as individuals in their own right (Heggestad et al., 2013).

Cohen-Mansfield and Jensen (2007) found that self-care habits and abilities change when a person with dementia moves into long-term care. They compared the changes seen in people with dementia attending day care and those in a nursing home and found that while the first group maintained their individual habits, those in the second group did not. Changes were seen in almost all aspects of daily routines, particularly around sleep, eating, dressing and bathing. It was not clear from the research what the main causes of these changes were. These findings would seem to indicate that the transition to the care home did not enable people living with dementia to retain some of their basic activities of daily living skills.

Change is difficult for many people in many situations, however moving into a care home is perhaps one of the most difficult transitions to navigate for both the person living with dementia and their family. Care homes have many different approaches to improving the care experience for residents, and it is not our purpose in this book to discuss this. We are drawing attention to the evidence that suggests that moving into a care home is rarely perceived as a positive choice, rather it is a decision that has to be made in often very difficult circumstances.

CHAPTER SUMMARY

In this chapter we have looked at the transitions that occur as the person living with dementia has increased care needs or the person providing support may no longer be able to provide the support they once did, this may mean more community-based support, or a stay in a hospital or move to a care home. We have seen that accepting the need for increased care and support is difficult for family members and the person living with dementia and it requires a sensitive and sympathetic approach from professionals and practitioners. Family members can experience combinations of grief, guilt, relief or sorrow and people with dementia can experience disorientation, losses and anxiety. The need for increased support can sometimes be due to symptoms changing and care needs developing, and the person may continue to live well with dementia at home. However, over time, increased care support needs often lead to end of life care. It is to this issue that we turn in chapter 7.

REFERENCES

Adams, K.B. and Sanders, S. (2004) Alzheimer's caregiver differences in experience of loss, grief reactions and depressive symptoms across stage of disease: A mixed method analysis. *Dementia* 3(2):195–210. doi: 10.1177/1471301204042337

Afram, B., Verbeek, H., Bleijlevens, M.H.C. and Hamers, J.P.H. (2015) Needs of informal caregivers during transition from home towards institutional care in dementia: A systematic review of qualitative studies. *International Psychogeriatrics* 27(6):891–902. doi: 10.1017/S1041610214002154

Alzheimer Disease International (2016) *World Alzheimer Report 2016 Improving Healthcare for People Living with Dementia Coverage, Quality and Costs Now and in the Future.* www.alz.co.uk/research/World AlzheimerReport2016.pdf

Alzheimer Society (2009) *Counting the Cost: Caring for People with Dementia on Hospital Wards.* London. www.alzheimers.org.uk/ sites/default/files/2018-05/Counting_the_cost_report.pdf

Blandin, K. and Pepin, R. (2017) Dementia grief: A theoretical model of a unique grief experience. *Dementia* 16(1):67–78. doi: 10.1177/1471301215581081

Briggs, R., Coary, R., Collins, R., Coughlan, T., O'Neill, D. and Kennelly, S.P. (2015) Acute hospital care: How much activity is attributable to caring for patients with dementia? *Quarterly Journal Medicine* 109(1):41–44.

Caron, C.D., Ducharme, F. and Griffith, J. (2006) Deciding on institutionalisation for a relative with dementia: The most difficult decision for caregivers. *Canadian Journal on Aging* 25:193–205. doi: 10.1353/cja.2006.003316821201

Chang, Y.-P., Kraenzle Schneider, J. and Sessanna, L. (2011) Decisional conflict among Chinese family caregivers regarding nursing home placement of older adults with dementia. *Journal of Aging Studies* 25:436–444. doi: 10.1016/j.jaging.2011.05.001

Cheung, D.S.K., Ho, K.H.M., Cheung, T.F., Lam, S.C. and Tse, M.M.Y. (2018) Anticipatory grief of spousal and adult children caregivers of people with dementia. *BMC Palliative Care*. doi: 10.1186/s12904-018-0376-3

Cho, S., Zarit, S.H. and Chiriboga, D.A. (2009) Wives and daughters: The differential role of day care use in the nursing home placement of cognitively impaired family members. *The Gerontologist* 49(1):57–67. doi: 10.1093/geront/gnp010

Cohen-Mansfield, J. and, Jensen, B. (2007) Changes in habits related to self-care in dementia: The nursing home versus adult day care. *American Journal of Alzheimer's Disease & Other Dementias*. doi.org/10.1177/1533317507301589

Department of Health (2009) *Living Well with Dementia: A National Dementia Strategy*. London; Department of Health. www.iow.nhs.uk/uploads/General/pdfs/Living%20well%20with%20dementia%20-%20a%20National%20Dementia%20Strategy%20-%20Accessible%20Summary.pdf

Dewing, J. and Dijk, S. (2016) What is the current state of care for older people with dementia in general hospitals? A literature review. *Dementia* 15(1):106–124.

Dickinson, D., Bamford, C., Exley, C., Emmett, C., Hughes, J. and Louise Robinson, L. (2013) Planning for tomorrow whilst living for today: The views of people with dementia and their families on advance care planning. *International Psychogeriatrics* 25(12):2011–2021. doi: 10.1017/S1041610213001531

Edvardsson, D. and Nordvall, K. (2008) Lost in the present but confident of the past: Experiences of being in a psycho-geriatric unit as narrated by persons with dementia. *Journal of Clinical Nursing* 17(4):491–498. doi: 10.1111/j.1365-2702.2006.01826.x

Featherstone, K., Northcott, A. and Bridges, J. (2019) Routines of resistance: An ethnography of the care of people living with dementia in acute hospital wards and its consequences. *International Journal of Nursing Studies* 96:53–60. doi: 10.1016/j.ijnurstu.2018.12.009

Graneheim, U.H., Johansson, A. and Lindgren, B.M. (2014) Family caregivers' experiences of relinquishing the care of a person with dementia to a nursing home: Insights from a meta-ethnographic study. *Scandanavian Journal of Caring Science* 28:215–224.

Haesler, E., Bauer, M. and Nay, R. (2007) Staff-family relationships in the care of older people: A report on a systematic review. *Research in Nursing and Health* 30:385–398.

Heggestad, A.K.T., Nortvedt, P. and Slettebø, A. (2013) "Like a prison without bars": Dementia and experiences of dignity. *Nursing Ethics* 20(8):881–892. doi:10.1177/0969733013484484

Innes, A., Abela, S. and Scerri, C. (2011) The organisation of dementia care by families in Malta: The experiences of family caregivers. *Dementia* 10(2):165–184.

Innes, A., Kelly, F. and Dincarslan, O. (2011) Care home design for people with dementia: What do people with dementia and their family carers value? *Aging & Mental Health* 15(5):548–556.

Innes, A., Kelly, F., Scerri, C. and Abela, S. (2016) Living with dementia in hospital wards: A comparative study of staff perceptions of practice and observed patient experience. *International Journal Nursing Older People*. doi: 10.1111/opn.12102

Kelley, R., Godfrey, M. and Young, J. (2019) The impacts of family involvement on general hospital care experiences for people living with dementia: An ethnographic study. *International Journal of Nursing Studies* 96:72–81. doi.org/10.1016/j.ijnurstu.2019.04.004

Lord, K., Livingston, G. and Cooper, C. (2015) A systematic review of barriers and facilitators to and interventions for proxy decision-making by family carers of people with dementia. *International Psychogeriatrics* 27(8):1301–1312.

Lord, K., Livingston, G., Robertson, S. and Cooper, C. (2016) How people with dementia and their families decide about moving to a care home and support their needs: Development of a decision aid, a qualitative study. *BMC Geriatrics* 16:68. doi: 10.1186/s12877-016-0242-1

MacCourt, P., McLennan, M., Somers, S. and Krawczyk, M. (2017) Effectiveness of a grief intervention for caregivers of people with dementia. *Omega (Westport)* 75(3):230–247. doi: 10.1177/0030222816652802

Moon, H., Dilworth-Anderson, P. and Gräske, J. (2017) The effects of placement on dementia care recipients' and family caregivers' quality of life: A literature review. *Quality in Ageing Older Adults* 18(1):44–57.

Moyle, W., Borbasi, S., Wallis, M., Olorenshaw, R. and Gracia, N. (2011) Acute care management of older people with dementia: A qualitative perspective. *Journal of Clinical Nursing* 20(3–4):420–428.

National Institute Care Excellence (NICE) (2019) *Delirium*: Prevention, diagnosis and management. *Clinical Guideline [CG103]*. Published date: July 2010. www.nice.org.uk/guidance/cg103/chapter/Introduction [accessed March 2019].

Nay, R. (1996) Relatives' experiences of nursing homelife: Characterised by tension. *Australasian Journal on Ageing* 16:24–29.

O'Reilly, J. and Shatz, R. (2019) *Dementia and Alzheimer's: Solving the Practical and Policy Challenges*. London, UK and New York, NY, USA: Anthem Press. doi: 10.2307/j.ctvg5bsr1

Owen, L.G. and Dening, K.H. (2018) Exploring therapeutic interventions to reduce the experience of guilt in carers of people living with dementia. *British Journal of Neuroscience* 14(6):286–291. doi: 10.12968/bjnn.2018.14.6.286

Parke, B., Hunter, K.F., Strain, L.A., Marck, P.B., Waugh, E.H. and McClelland, A.J. (2013) Facilitators and barriers to safe emergency department transitions for community dwelling older people with dementia and their caregivers: A social ecological study. *International Journal of Nursing Studies* 50(9):1206–1218.

Porock, D., Clissett, P., Harwood, R. and Gladman, J. (2015) Disruption, control and coping: Responses of and to the person with dementia in hospital. *Ageing and Society* 35(1):37–63.

Rosén, H., Behm, L., Wallerstedt, B. and Ahlstrom, G. (2019) Being the next of kin of an older person living in a nursing home: An interview study about quality of life. *BMC Geriatrics* 19:324. doi:10.1186/s12877-019-1343-4

Sampson, E.L., Blanchard, M.R., Jones, L., Tookman, A. and King, M. (2009) Dementia in the acute hospital: Prospective cohort study of prevalence and mortality. *British Journal of Psychiatry* 195(1):61–66.

Sampson, E.L., Leurent, B., Blanchard, M.R., Jones, L. and King, M. (2013) Survival of people with dementia after unplanned acute hospital admission: A prospective cohort study. *International Journal of Geriatric Psychiatry* 28(10):1015–1022.

Scerri, A., Innes, A. and Scerri, C. (2017) Dementia training programmes for staff working in general hospital settings: A systematic review of the literature. *Aging and Mental Health* 21(8):783–796. doi: 10.1080/13607863.2016.1231170

Scerri, A., Scerri, C. and Innes, A. (2018) The perceived and observed needs of patients with dementia admitted to acute medical wards. *Dementia*. doi: 10.1177/1471301218814383

Tatangelo, G., McCabe, M., Macleod, A. and Konis, A. (2018) "I just can't please them all and stay sane": Adult child caregivers' experiences of family dynamics in care- giving for a parent with dementia in Australia. *Health and Social Care in the Community* 26(3):370–377. doi: 10.1111/hsc.12534

Walker, R.J. and Pomeroy, E.C. (1997) The impact of anticipatory grief on caregivers of persons with Alzheimer's disease. *Home Health Care Service Quarterly* 16(1–2):55–76. doi: 10.1300/ J027v16n01_05

Woods, R.T., Keady, J. and Seddon, D. (2008) *Involving Families in Care Homes: A Relationship-Centred Approach to Dementia Care.* London: Jessica Kingsley.

7

END OF LIFE CARE

This chapter considers what is often the most difficult time in the journey with dementia, that is, the time leading up to, and the death of the person with, dementia. In 2008 (Department of Health), the first national strategy for end of life care commissioned in England highlighted three specific problems:

1 that people did not die in their place of choice;
2 that health care providers needed to prepare for larger numbers of people dying; and
3 that the quality of care was not equal.

Since then policy directives around good end of life/palliative care have developed (both in the UK and internationally). However as Sampson et al. (2011) note, although policy and guidelines abound, there is still much to be done to ensure that end of life care improves in practice for people living with dementia and their families. Person-centred care at end of life has taken greater focus (Lloyd-Williams et al., 2017), with key principles of ensuring that individual needs are met, taking into consideration how the person wants to be cared for, where they want to be cared for, where they wish to die and their spiritual and religious needs.

The crucial role of family members in the care of people who are terminally ill has been acknowledged, particularly where there is a lack of formal services available (Burns et al., 2013). Family members helping with the care of people towards the end of their life may be children, grandchildren, spouses or in-laws, and each will have different experiences of caring for the person with dementia, depending on their physical proximity, resources, care roles and existing relationship with the person and other family members (Small et al., 2007). Decision making at end of life can be challenging for family members if advance care planning has not been carried out and the person with dementia was not consulted about their wishes when they had the ability to contribute to decision making. The importance of having the conversations around dying and death at an early point in the journey with dementia, rather than when the person is considered to be at end of life cannot be overstated; the resource produced by TIDE and DEEP (2018) provides ideas and tips on how to have these conversations and talk about end of life preferences. This is a real change in how end of life care is approached in dementia and provides clear evidence of the increasing focus on end of life care over the last 15 or so years. Guidelines exist for practitioners to refer to as they work with an individual living with dementia and their family members in providing support when they are at end of life (e.g. North West Coast Strategic Clinical Network, 2018; National Council for Palliative Care Dementia, 2014). These guidelines are accessible and useful for family members as well as professionals as they navigate what is often one of the most difficult periods of dementia care.

WHAT DO WE MEAN BY END OF LIFE CARE?

The term end of life care is generally applied to those who are approaching death. This is a time when it is assumed that the person does not have long to live, the prognosis for recovery is not good and there is little that can be done in terms of treatment. The aim moves from ensuring quality of life to ensuring a comfortable death, by finding ways to make the person comfortable and attending to their needs and wishes as the end of their life approaches.

There have been clear intentions stated for over a decade now that all people approaching the end of life, regardless of age, diagnosis, gender, ethnicity, sexual orientation, religious belief, disability or socio-economic status (Department of Health, 2008), should receive high-quality care whether they are at home, in a care home, hospice, hospital or elsewhere. People living with dementia and their family members can expect that end of life care will be high quality and they will receive support appropriate to their particular needs.

The foundations of end of life dementia care are built on the aims of the Department of Health (2008, 17–18) End of Life Care Strategy, which stated that people will have:

- The opportunity to discuss their personal needs with professionals who can support them and the opportunity to have these needs and preferences recorded in a care plan.
- Coordinated care and support, ensuring that their needs are met, irrespective of who is delivering the service.
- Rapid specialist advice and clinical assessment, wherever the person lives.
- High-quality care and support during the last days of life.
- Services which treat people with dignity and respect before and after death.
- Ongoing appropriate advice and support for carers.

With such high expectations for care, it is vital that staff are well trained, particularly in communication skills, and have a good understanding of the needs of all concerned: the person with dementia, that is, their patient, the family members and others involved in the care of the person.

It can be difficult to decide at what point the care of a person with dementia becomes 'end of life' care, particularly as the life expectancy of people with dementia has grown over time even when their dementia is deemed to be quite 'advanced'. A further difficulty arises from negative assumptions about dementia (McParland et al., 2017), including the old but still commonly used description that dementia can be a 'living death' and so all dementia care could be seen as end of life care. Clearly such negative assumptions about dementia do little to create a caring environment where the potential of each person is maximised, even as death approaches. There are, however, particular challenges in deciding at what point in time death is approaching for the person with dementia and when appropriate care should be provided.

WHAT IS PALLIATIVE CARE?

The understanding of the nature and purpose of palliative care has changed over time – previous understandings of palliative care viewed its instigation once cure is no longer feasible, whereas current understandings see supportive and palliative care instigated at diagnosis and increasing up to, and beyond, death. Thus, palliative care is not just about care in the last months, days and hours of a person's life, but about ensuring quality of life for the person living with dementia and their families at every point of the process from diagnosis onwards. Palliative and end of life care are now seen as integral aspects of the care delivered by any health or social care professional to those living with and dying from any advanced, progressive or incurable condition, including dementia.

The Social Care Institute for Excellence (2015) has an online guide that discusses key issues relating to end of life care in dementia. This is an excellent resource that draws on the developments made in the dementia care field over the last decade or so. Palliative care is about ensuring quality of life and comfort up until the point of death. It considers four elements key to good end of life care:

- Pain control.
- Eating and drinking at end of life.
- End of life care needs and the needs of the care supporters.
- Care in the last days and hours of a person's life.

These issues have been reported widely in the literature as challenges for both professionals and family members in different settings, whether this be at home or in care homes or hospitals (Miranda et al., 2019; Glass, 2016).

WHERE DO PEOPLE DIE?

Remaining at home may be the preferred option for family carers and the person with dementia (Goodman et al., 2010; Hirakawa et al., 2006), however evidence suggests that people do not always have their preferences met. The National End of Life Care Intelligence Network briefing (2016) documents where people with dementia commonly die:

> The place of death profile for people who have died with dementia is markedly different compared with the general population. For those aged 65+, the majority of deaths with a mention of dementia occurred in care homes (58%), nearly a third of deaths in hospitals and less than a tenth at home. In contrast, in the general population aged 65+, nearly half of all deaths occurred in hospitals, a quarter in care homes and one fifth at home. A very small proportion of people who have died with dementia do so in hospices (1%) compared with the general population (5%).
>
> (2016, 4)

The reality, in the UK, is that few people with advanced and complex dementia die at home, and few live at home in the months leading up to the end of their lives. This may be because family carers are not equipped to deal with increasing levels of agitation, depression or behaviour disturbances, which may occur as dementia progresses. However, although providing end of life care for someone with dementia can be desirable and successful for some, it is not always feasible. Nursing care may be required or other specialist health and social care input that often requires a co-coordinated and multi-disciplinary approach.

One of the Alzheimer Society's (2012) seven recommendations in relation to end of life care for people living with dementia relates to place of death. They recommend that:

> People with dementia at the end of their lives should be able to access high-quality services to meet their needs at any time of the day or night regardless of the setting. They argue that people living with dementia 'should have a holistic needs assessment', and that Commissioners should commission services that enable people with dementia to be cared for where they want to be at the end of their lives. This includes commissioning for community and care home settings and considering different models of care that meet the needs of people with dementia throughout the course of their illness.
>
> (2012, 27)

However, recommendations do not always relate to the lived experiences of people living with dementia and their families.

Dying at home

Understandably, most people living with dementia and their family members wish for the person to be able to live at home until they die and seek ways of enabling this to happen (Small et al., 2007; Lloyd–Williams et al., 2017). This is not without its difficulties as there may be limited support available and the challenges of providing end of life care can be considerable (Miranda et al., 2019), mentally, emotionally, financially and practically.

Gail's story of caring for her mother at home until her death

> To everything there is a season,
> And a time for every matter under heaven,
> A time to be born and a time to die . . .

Book of Ecclesiastes

These lines from the Bible show the frailty of human life. We are all born so inevitably we will all die. Talking about end of life is not easy, but it is one common denominator we all possess. Having lived through the experience of losing my mother to non-Parkinson's dementia with Lewy bodies and experiencing my father being placed on the end of life pathway with mixed cortex, sub-cortical vascular dementia, it is my hope that by sharing my experience it will belie any myths that surround end stage dementia, including end of life care; and that it will provide the reader with sound practical advice regarding hospital admissions, palliative care, end of life support and bereavement.

I have experienced reluctance from professionals to start the difficult conversations early enough so that the person with dementia can take part in advance care planning. My mother was never asked by professionals what her thoughts were regarding her own care, but I ensured we had that important conversation. Upon diagnosis my mother was already perceived as 'too severe'. Doctors felt she lacked capacity to decide for herself how and where she would like to be cared for and consequently where she would like to die. In England, if a person with dementia is deemed severe, then under the Mental Capacity Act (2005) decisions about care are taken away from them under deprivation of liberty (DoL). Luckily, my mother and I had already had a conversation about her wishes many years before. I therefore knew that my mother did not want to be placed into a care home, nor did she like hospitals, and that when the time came she would like to die at home, in her own surroundings and with those who loved her. She was a very pragmatic and intelligent lady, with a strong will and great determination. Yet, even though I conveyed her wishes as her power of attorney, when the time arose, I was still 'advised' to put my mother into a care home, as it would be 'better for all concerned'.

My mother had said to me, 'None of us can live forever, but I will live my life how I want, and I will die on my own terms'.

I wanted to support her to do this and nursed my mother at home until the very end.

From my own experience, when my mother's dementia progressed to end stage, I saw a decline in her overall health. She became more susceptible to infections and lost the ability to swallow properly. She also had cancer for the last 18 months of her life, which in itself added further complications. Our situation was different to some as the decision was to nurse mum at home. As a carer I knew that I needed to look at what support was available and how to access this. I found that the district nurses become invaluable, especially if you build a rapport with your named nurse. I also found that the community psychiatric nurse (CPN) was like an angel throughout those gruelling months. Our situation meant that my mother required palliative care. We had an assessment from the MacMillan nursing team; however, we were declined support from this service as we already had district nurse intervention. Though we did not have the support from MacMillan on a daily basis, they did authorise a grant that would help us to purchase a special reclining chair. This chair proved vital in the later stages of my mother's illness, ensuring her comfort especially when she didn't want to sleep in her bed. All cases are assessed individually, so support is tailored to suit the situation.

I am still going through my own bereavement two years since my mother passed. I know how hard it is to get on with living, the emptiness that can consume you, but I also know that I am not alone, and that I have great peer support – which is the most valuable asset I have.

HOSPITALS AND END OF LIFE CARE

Often before a person is entered onto an end of life pathway, they will have been admitted into hospital. Establishing appropriate and effective end of life pathways has been recognised as a key component of good quality care. One of the most popular tools practitioners used in hospitals (although it was also used in other settings) up until the last 10 years was the Liverpool Care Pathway; however this was heavily critiqued and then withdrawn, resulting in practitioners reporting a loss of confidence in approaching end of life care (Torjesen, 2013). There are many different frameworks and models (Kumar and Kuriakose, 2013); one of the most popular and used approaches is the Gold Standards Framework.

Gold Standards Framework

The Gold Standards Framework (GSF) was originally developed in 2000 as an initiative to improve palliative care within primary care. Full information about this framework can be found at www.goldstandardsframework.org.uk/.

It is one of the most developed models of end of life care. It enables those approaching the end of life to be identified, their care needs assessed and a plan of care developed and put in place with all relevant agencies. The framework focuses on optimising continuity of care, teamwork, advanced planning (including out of hours), symptom control and patient, carer and staff support. Although developed for use in primary care, it can be used in all care settings.

The GSF has five goals:

1   The right care at the right time for the right person.
2   Care that is person-centred and carer-centred.
3   Care that plans ahead rather than simply reacting in an emergency or critical situation.
4   Care closer to where the person with dementia wants to be cared for and to reduce unnecessary admissions to hospital.
5   Partnerships working so that the person with dementia receives good care in all care settings.

SCIE (2015)

These translate into seven key tasks:

1   Communication.
2   Co-ordination.
3   Control of symptoms.
4   Continuity of care.

5   Carer support.
6   Care of dying pathway.
7   Continued learning.

The GSF is used to support the end of life care needs of people with dementia in care homes (GSFCH) and has five key themes:

1   Pre-planning – including needs-based coding of all residents and linking with the needs support matrices, advance care planning discussions offered to *all* residents as standard practice, better pre-emptive planning with GPs, anticipatory prescribing, out of hours handover forms and pathways/protocols for care in the final days.
2   Improved communication – listening to peoples' real concerns and needs, talking more easily about the subject of care towards the end of life, communicating better with others and improved means of written documentation.
3   Improved team-work and collaboration both within the home and between others in the community, for example, with GPs, hospice/palliative care, primary care trusts and local authorities.
4   Decreasing hospitalisation – by reducing avoidable hospital admissions and leading to more people dying with dignity in the home, improving hospital turnaround of patients to facilitate an earlier discharge.
5   High-quality clinical care, with good assessment and management of symptoms, identifying specific needs of those with dementia and the prevention of avoidable crises.

Research comparing end of life practices in care homes in which the GSFCH was implemented and those in which it was not, Badger et al. (2009) found that homes that used the programme reported significant improvements in processes to identify and address the needs of residents with end of life care needs. They also reported a reduction in the number of crisis admissions to hospital and a significant increase in the percentage of residents who died in a care home rather than a hospital. Although collaboration with other professionals is important, the strength of the GSF is its emphasis on encouraging 'Gold Standard' thinking throughout the entire care setting.

Pathways in practice

Working within these pathways to promote quality of life can be difficult for health and social care professionals who work with people with dementia, as they challenge long-held assumptions about inevitable decline and lack of quality of life as dementia progresses. There are many challenges to improving end of life care for people with dementia and their families, including unrealistic expectations regarding prognosis, continued non-recognition of pain in people with dementia who are dying and finding a balance between over- and under-treating (Thune-Boyle et al., 2010). Davies et al. (2018) discuss the development and use of heuristics, that is, a set of common principles, to aid practitioners in end of life dementia care. This approach developed guides for four challenges commonly identified as difficult for practitioners: eating and swallowing; agitation/restlessness; reviewing treatment and interventions at the end of life; and providing routine care at the end of life. This work is new but offers the opportunity to develop guidelines that will work in practice for practitioners as they think through 'in the moment' decision making while working to support people living with dementia at end of life. The Alzheimer Society (2012) have recommended that hospital staff and staff in all settings receive the appropriate support and training to enable them to deliver high-quality end of life care. In their review of the research around end of life dementia care in hospitals Moon et al. (2018) found that people with dementia were less likely to receive aggressive interventions but that the provision of end of life care symptom management was not adequate generally. This suggests that end of life care in hospitals and other settings will continue to be an area of research enquiry, as although there are policies, guidelines and principles that seek to enhance end of life care, the reality may not be the same in practice.

Gail's experience when her father, Ron, was in hospital

I was challenged on numerous occasions about my presence on the ward outside of normal visiting times. Often it was due to a lack of understanding by ward staff about John's Campaign, a locally developed guide based on local experiences; others just felt that I was in the way. However, I was an extra pair of hands, especially at meal times. I also took care of all the personal care needs my father had and I was the constant he required. My father also has separation anxiety, which is part of his dementia. My presence reduced his distress and orientated him, thus reducing delirium. Whilst in hospital, my father was put on the end of life pathway. The reason was that the clinicians felt that he displayed hypoactive delirium, frailty, mixed morbidity and he was losing weight. However, the hypoactive delirium was just my father wanting to sleep and get himself well, something he has always done. The frailty is due to the numerous infections he had to battle, the mixed morbidity he has lived with for many years, and losing weight was due to my father not liking hospital food!

A GOOD DEATH?

A common aspect of end of life and palliative care is to provide a 'good death'. What this means to different people can vary, however there are common components that have been identified (Small et al., 2007, 180):

- Facing death in which the person is aware and accepting of impending death.
- Preparations for death in which the person considers the rituals he/she wants, completes his/her worldly affairs and makes plans for dying.
- Environmental preparations in which the person considers different aspects of the environment in which death takes place, including the degree of technology involved and the extent to which death can be peaceful.

However, there are possible tensions here, between the person who is dying, his/her family and staff involved in the care of the person. The person may prioritise awareness, the relatives or staff pain control or the control of symptoms. What about the person who has ceased to be aware and is unable to make final preparations: are they excluded from this category of people who can aspire to a good death? Small et al. (2007) have argued that, traditionally, a palliative care approach has not engaged with the needs of people with dementia who are dying, because palliative care has at its core autonomy and choice, not always accessible to people with dementia who are dying. However, they argue that excellent palliative care and excellent dementia care can each add richness to the other approach. The contribution that palliative care could make to dementia care includes:

- Its expertise in technical and procedural skills.
- Its optimism.
- Its focus on forward planning and consultation.

The contribution of excellent dementia care to palliative care includes:

- Its multi-disciplinary approach in responding to multiple pathologies.
- The development of longer-term relationships with people with dementia and their families.
- Expertise in engaging with people who have limited or no verbal abilities.
- Expertise in working with cognitive and behavioural changes.

Research has become more concerned about the perceptions of families in terms of good-quality end of life care (Mogan et al., 2018). An early review of eight studies looking at family members' views of end of life care for people living with dementia found that there was more variance in terms of care preferences than similarities in end of life experiences (Davies et al., 2014). More recent UK research found (Davies et al., 2017) that family members perceived that maintaining the person within, preserving respect and dignity and showing compassion and kindness were key to quality end of life care. Dutch research (De Roo et al., 2014) investigated both the number of residents and the circumstances in which residents of long-term care facilities die peacefully. Peaceful death was seen in relation to personal factors, but also emotional and spiritual care needs. They found that of the 233 residents in their study, 56 percent were perceived by their family members to have had a peaceful death. The availability of some form of spiritual care and involvement in decision making were seen as key elements that contributed to a peaceful death.

What constitutes dying well with dementia from the perspective of the person with dementia has rarely been examined. Hill et al.

(2017) investigated what people living with dementia and their families thought was important about end of life care. They found a lack of consensus as to what was most important, demonstrating that end of life care, as with all dementia care, needs to be individualised and take account of the individual and their family's preferences and needs. The areas of consensus they did identify related to wanting more information and more involvement in decision making (rather than professionals making all the decisions) and for compassionate care to be given when the person was approaching the end of their life.

A very stark expectation of a good death has been presented by Lawrence et al. (2011) as simply a death free from pain. This may seem a very basic principle but ascertaining if someone with dementia is in pain can be very difficult when verbal communication is limited.

Lesley's view on end of life

When my life is nearing its end I have spoken quite a lot to my family and friends about what I would like to happen, whilst I have capacity to make my own decisions.

Life is just a journey and I want mine to be as smooth as possible for me and my family. I don't want resuscitating, I don't want feeding with a tube or peg feeding; I would like my mouth kept moist and clean but that is all.

I want to live in my own home in familiar surroundings.

I know people find this difficult to comprehend but it should be my choice. Speaking, even to doctors, whilst I have capacity has been hard for them to understand and this shouldn't be the case.

I *never* want to go into a care or nursing home. Just let me go peacefully at home knowing you have fulfilled my wishes. The professionals must remember that just because I have dementia doesn't mean I can't feel pain. Look for the nonverbal signs that I am in pain and treat me like you would treat a cancer patient who can speak and tell you they have pain.

Having been with my husband at the end of his life I know how hard this can be for the family, but I fulfilled his wishes by keeping him in the house he loved with me until the time he died.

Dementia is like any other disease; it progresses and has an outcome – this outcome is death. When the time comes I won't be afraid, I will be released and set free.

ADVANCE DIRECTIVES OR ADVANCE CARE PLANS

Advance directives or advance care plans (ACP) can address ethical concerns and dilemmas inherent in decision-making at end of life. Here, the person living with dementia and often his/her family will document preferences for future health care, sometimes in collaboration with other health care professionals. This document is then kept for future reference, once the person with dementia is no longer able to be consulted about his/her wishes and preferences for care.

The advantages and disadvantages of advance directives can be summarised as follows.

Advantages

- Encourages communication about end of life decisions.
- Give directions to treatment decisions when the person is no longer able to decide for themselves.
- The person's autonomy is respected.

Disadvantages

- An individual may change their mind about what they want.
- Advance directives can be difficult to interpret.
- Can provoke anxiety for the person and their family.

They do however provide a way of trying to capture the individual's views on their preferred care at end of life. It is important that advance directives are drawn up while the person still understands the diagnosis, prognosis and options for care (Pinch, 2004), and that they are regularly reviewed (Nuffield Council on Bioethics, 2009).

In their review of advance care plans, Dening et al. (2011) found little evidence of people living with dementia having plans, and when they did exist it was not clear if having one made any difference in practice.

In a survey of care homes in the UK to study their advance care planning practices, Froggatt et al. (2008) found that while consultation about general care was undertaken in a majority of care homes, there was much less consistency in completing ACPs. While staff were trained in areas such as palliative and bereavement care, few had training in advance care planning. Difficulties in the ACP process included lack of staff confidence in broaching the subject and difficulties with ascertaining the resident's wishes. Although the study included care homes where people with dementia lived, this group of people generally appeared to be excluded in the ACP process, due in part to communication difficulties and managers' perceptions of lack of competency to make decisions.

In a recent review of 84 studies, Sellars et al. (2019) found that people living with dementia were uncertain about decisions they had to make for ACPs and that families and people living with dementia found it emotionally difficult to discuss issues relating to end of life. If plans were not in place family members found it difficult to liaise with health professionals later on regarding the best decision. This review demonstrates the ongoing complexities experienced by people living with dementia and their families in relation to ACPs and the support they require to both initially develop a plan and how to later implement decisions in light of the presence or absence of previously articulated wishes.

Decision making and the family

Whether or not there has been advance care planning discussions and documentation, issues and decisions that family members are asked to make that have been reported as difficult are:

- Whether or not to actively treat severe dehydration or infection.
- Whether or not to resuscitate.
- Whether deception or coercion to solve problems is justified.
- Balancing conflicts between the wishes and needs of different parties.
- Balancing invasive treatments with quality of life.
- How to know when the person is communicating and what they are communicating.
- When and how to prepare an advance directive or living will and whether this will be adhered to in the future.

When facing decisions such as these after perhaps providing support for many years, it is not surprising that family members commonly report experiencing guilt at some point throughout their caring role, but particularly at end of life. Family members may ask themselves, have I done enough? Could I have done things differently? Why did I put mum/dad/partner into a care home? The anger, frustration, isolation and loneliness of being a carer are a well-documented part of the journey as we have discussed throughout this book. They are all part of the grieving process too. Watching the person with dementia progress to end of life care can feel like a living bereavement.

Therefore, although advance care plans offer the opportunity to guide end of life care decision making and delivery, not enough people have them and even when they do exist, they have been found to be difficult to implement in practice. This can lead to challenges for those who have to make decisions about end of life care.

COMMON CHALLENGES IN PROVIDING HIGH-QUALITY END OF LIFE DEMENTIA CARE

There are many challenges that arise when providing support to someone at the end of life, however two particular challenges have been extensively and repeatedly examined: pain control and interventions in drinking and eating. We will briefly consider each in turn.

Pain control in dementia care

One of the consequences of maintaining people at home for as long as possible is that people admitted into hospital or a care home are generally quite frail, and many of them may have other age-related conditions. One of the areas that care staff and families need to be conscious of is recognising and managing pain. A review of studies of pain and dementia found that recognising distress associated with pain can be difficult, particularly when the person with dementia has difficulty communicating verbally (McAuliffe et al., 2012). Pain may be shown through signs of distress such as withdrawal and silence, reduction in activity, restlessness or aggression. In dementia care, if such behaviour is attributed to dementia, as opposed to other possible factors, the person's pain is at risk of being ignored (Small et al., 2007). Even if care staff or family members think that the person is in pain, they may find it difficult to work out what is wrong and how to help (Brorson et al., 2014).

Most assessment of pain relies on the ability of the person experiencing pain to report and describe their pain. However, people with dementia with communicative, reasoning and memory difficulties are harder to assess through verbal self-reporting, as they are less likely to be able to articulate where the pain is, what type of pain it is, how severe it is or how long it has been present. In practice, where there are difficulties in assessing pain, this is likely to lead to subsequent difficulties in managing pain (Horgas et al., 2007). Even if care professionals' sense that the person is in distress, they often lack a means of articulating or documenting that distress, and this can result in distress often going unmet as pain scales and assessments are often not adequate (Brown, 2011).

It is important that practitioners are aware of the different ways of evaluating pain. Horgas et al. (2007) evaluated the reliability and validity of a pain assessment tool called the Non-communicative Patient's Pain Assessment Instrument (NOPPAIN). NOPPAIN was developed to assess pain in non-communicative nursing home residents with advanced dementia. It uses six pain-related behaviours:

- Pain words.
- Pain noises.
- Pain faces.
- Rubbing.
- Bracing.
- Restlessness.

along with two dimensions of pain:

- Presence (yes or no).
- Intensity (rated from 0–5).

Horgas et al. (2007) found that the most common expressions of pain in those with cognitive impairment were facial expressions indicating pain, which they termed 'pain faces'. This highlights the important of observation skills and non-verbal communication awareness in those providing support to the person with dementia. The common elements that any pain assessment and management approach need to take into consideration are:

- Anticipate and assume the presence of pain resulting from disease, injury, procedure or surgery.

- Observe the person for behaviours to establish a baseline for subsequent behaviours. Monitor for pain regularly using a comprehensive list of pain-related behaviours (i.e. NOPPAIN). Ideally, do this during activity, as behaviour at rest may be misleading.
- Observe for less obvious indicators of pain, such as agitation, aggression or increased pacing.
- If the presence of pain is uncertain, an analgesic (pain relief) may be administered to evaluate the presence of pain. If the intervention appears to provide pain relief, pain may be assumed as the likely cause of the behaviour.

One of the seven recommendations from the UK Alzheimer Society (2012) relates specifically to pain. They argue that 'all people with dementia should be free from pain at the end of their lives, with training and systems designed to detect and manage pain even when communication is diminished' (2012, 8).

This brief overview demonstrates the complexity of effectively assessing and managing pain in end of life care of people with dementia. Pain management is a complex clinical process requiring thorough assessment, appropriate intervention and systematic reassessment (Horgas et al., 2007). The many tools in use, while not comprehensive or standardised, do have common principles and should be used in conjunction with observation, communication with family members and communication of findings with other staff members and draw on whatever knowledge of the person with dementia is possible (Wernham et al., 2018).

Artificial nutrition and hydration

One issue, which poses a particular challenge for staff and for the family, is whether or not to commence artificial feeding when a person with dementia is no longer able to swallow. However, there is very little evidence that artificial feeding or hydration improves or increases the quality of life of people living with dementia (Sampson et al., 2009).

Sometimes family members may wish to avail of life-prolonging treatment to 'hang on to' the person with dementia. This can be a difficult time for all concerned, and it can be an ethical dilemma as to whether or not to give the person artificial hydration and nutrition.

The Nuffield Council on Bioethics (2009, 4) suggests that:

> Good, ethical care recognises the value of the person with dementia. It aims to promote their wellbeing and autonomy. At the same time, it pays attention to the interests of carers who provide so much of the day-to-day support.

Arguments for the use of artificial nutrition and hydration include:

- Providing hydration and nutrition is a form of basic care that should not be denied to anyone.
- Allowing someone to die from thirst or starvation is inhumane.

Arguments against the use of artificial nutrition and hydration include:

- This type of care is invasive and disproportionate.
- Potential complications include infections, aspiration and fluid overload.
- No proven benefit.
- No proven discomfort in people who do not receive artificial feeding.

(Buiting et al., 2007)

People with dementia in long-term care are at risk of 'medicalised dying' if invasive interventions such as naso-gastric or percutaneous endoscopic gastric (PEG) tubes are used to deliver nutrition when the person has ceased to swallow (Dekkers, 2004, 116). Increasingly, palliative care of people with dementia seeks to maintain the 'naturalness of dying' (Dekkers, 2004, 129) and how this can be ethically achieved.

The UK Alzheimer Society has produced guidance on artificial feeding that is helpful for family members to read when they encounter this challenge: www.alzheimers.org.uk/get-support/daily-living/making-decisions-artificial-feeding.

CULTURAL DIFFERENCES IN END OF LIFE ISSUES

Different cultural groups will have different attitudes to aspects of palliative care. Food and pain control are two aspects which have the most impact on palliative care. For example, during Ramadan, strict

Muslims will refuse oral analgesia during the fasting period. Some will refuse intravenous analgesia, preferring instead to endure pain.

Not all social or cultural groups have the same response to pain. Pain may be seen as resulting from some transgression, in which case penitence is called for. Pain may also be perceived as a misfortune or as a punishment, in which case the person must endure it (Davis, 2007). When considering pain relief, this is important to bear in mind. An awareness of different cultural understandings of pain and its management will be invaluable when providing end of life care for people with dementia and in the emotional support given to family members at this time.

A knowledge of the different beliefs different people have may help in understanding the concerns and fears of family members when asking them to make end of life decisions. For example, in Chinese research on family caregivers of people with dementia in Hong Kong, Kwok et al. (2007) found that most family members would not want to forgo life-sustaining treatment, even if their relative was comatose. Also, Kwok et al. (2007) found that family caregivers lacked certainty about their decision and preferred to consult with others such as family, friends or GP before arriving at a decision. This may reflect the tendency in some Chinese families to make collective decisions.

In contrast, Jewish law not only permits, but requires, the cessation of life-prolonging treatment if this is just delaying the inevitable, even if this means that the person will die more quickly. Factors which aid in this decision include whether the person is suffering, the prognosis, the stated preference of the person and whether the treatment is seen as extraordinary. However, applying these principles to a person in the terminal stages of dementia may be more difficult as it may be hard to determine whether they are suffering and what their preferences would be. This means that each case is determined on an individual basis with an emphasis on preserving the dignity of the person (Jotkowitz et al., 2005).

In their review, Connelly et al. (2012) found that artificial nutrition was more common in African American and Asian groups, but that attitudes towards end of life were found to be more common between different ethnic and cultural groups. Therefore, bearing in mind differences is important, but the grief and confusion that surround end of life is universal.

CULTURAL DIFFERENCES IN DEALING WITH DEATH

Religious belief and practice is a wide-ranging and complex topic. This section provides the customs of five major world faiths regarding death, arranged in alphabetical order, as a starting point to think about spiritual and religious needs and preferences (Allen, 2002).

> *Christianity* – Prayers may be said at the point of death, with anointing and laying on of hands accompanying prayer. Prayers for the departed and for those who are bereaved along with pastoral support may be appropriate following death. Post-mortem and organ donation and cremation are acceptable to most Christians.
>
> *Hinduism* – Hindus cremate their dead and this ritual must be led by the oldest son, no matter how young he may be. Hindus like to put some water from the river Ganges in the dying person's mouth and to bring some money or material things to be touched by the dying person, in the knowledge that this is given to charity after their death. Post-mortem is accepted, although disliked. Hindus do not like the body to be touched by non-Hindus. The family will usually want to wash the body at home. All adult Hindus are cremated.
>
> *Islam* – When dying, the person's face should be turned towards Mecca and a chapter of the Qur'an recited. After death, the arms and legs should be straightened and the toes tied together by a thread, the mouth and eyes are closed, and clothes should be removed by a person of the same gender. After death, the body should be washed by someone of the same gender and it should not be touched by non-Muslims. If care staff must touch the body, they should wear disposable gloves. Traditional preparation of the body for burial is strictly observed and this should take place within 24 hours after death. Local mosques may have full facilities for preparing the body for burial. Muslims are always buried, never cremated. Post-mortem is forbidden, unless ordered by a coroner.
>
> *Judaism* – Prayers are said when dying. After death, the immediate family should be notified as soon as possible. The body should be handled as little as possible and burial should take place within 24 hours. Post-mortem is only allowed if there is a legal requirement. The orthodox and reformed Jews have

separate burial grounds. Orthodox Jews are always buried, while Reformed Jews may opt for cremation.

Sikhism – Sikhs strictly cremate their dead. A post-mortem is not acceptable unless it is legally unavoidable. Generally, Sikhs are happy for non-Sikhs to tend to the body, although many families may wish to wash and lay out the body themselves. Adult Sikhs are always cremated, which should take place as soon as possible after death.

Practical steps to take to ensure that religious customs are adhered to include:

- Asking the person with dementia, if this is possible.
- Asking relatives and friends.
- Looking in the local telephone directory for the nearest faith establishment.
- Contacting the chaplaincy at the local HNS Trust, via the switchboard, for advice on other faiths such as Buddhist, Baha'i, Chinese or Rastafarian faiths.

In their review of spirituality in intensive care units (ICUs), Ho et al. (2017) demonstrate that often the spiritual and religious needs of people at end of life are not taken into account, but provide examples of the benefits to the person and their families when care is taken to observe spiritual needs, such as increased perceptions of quality of care, less aggressive care interventions and greater family satisfaction with the care experience. Spirituality and feeling connected to something bigger than the current moment can provide families with a coping mechanism (Slape, 2014) during the last weeks, days and hours of the person with dementia's death. This clearly indicates the benefits of spiritual care but it is often overlooked.

Jolley et al.'s (2010) study of people with dementia and their carers' views of spirituality found that people with dementia found particular comfort from engaging in routines of spiritual practices and carers used spiritual practices as a coping support. Jolley et al. (2010) suggest that questions about spirituality and faith should form part of routine assessments, and care plans should be revised to accommodate identified or changing spiritual needs. This will bring dementia services into line with palliative care services.

Professional carers may develop deeply human relationships with those they care for and with family members, with all the potential difficulties that accompany them. This means considering the psychological, social and spiritual needs of individuals during their entire journey with dementia (Small et al., 2007), and not just at the terminal stage.

If we are truly to address end of life care for people with dementia, it is essential that those who provide such care are well supported to enable them to engage with the emotional world of the person with dementia as death approaches.

BEREAVEMENT

Inevitably, death will occur at some point along the dementia journey. Bereavement is as unique to an individual as a fingerprint, as we all mourn differently and for varying lengths of time. This can be due to religious or cultural beliefs, how close we were to the person who has died and how much support we receive. One thing that we should not forget is that professional care providers also need to grieve, especially if they have been involved in the care of the person for a long time. Many feel that they have closure if they are invited to the funeral or to memorial services. Even though they are professionals, they are still human.

A common theme that is evident is a sense of relief. Relief is not a selfish feeling, but a pragmatic one. The relief is that now the person with the dementia is free. Free from being locked into an alien world, free from fear and agitation and free from any pain they may have had towards the end. Carers should not feel guilty for this feeling.

Family members may also find that once their caring role ends that they have to adjust and 're-find themselves'. This is common, as many family members give up their careers, hobbies and other interests to look after their loved one on a full-time basis. It is easy to lose confidence, particularly if you need to re-enter into work. Bereavement support will help with this.

The following are a few tips for when a person dies:

- Avoid making any hasty decisions, such as moving to a new house.
- Keep items that were important to the person – this may help you to stay connected.

- Seek support so that you are not isolated.
- Note that it is not unusual to think that you hear their voice or smell their perfume/aftershave.
- Look after your own spiritual needs.
- Look for support from bereavement services if you feel that you are overwhelmed.

DYING AND DEATH – THOSE LEFT BEHIND

The death of a family member, particularly after a long illness, can be distressing for those left behind. Although family members may report levels of stress and burden, they can demonstrate remarkable resilience after the death of a person with dementia. Watching a loved one slowly die is not only distressing, but can also raise feelings of anger, guilt and powerlessness.

It is perhaps unsurprising that there is less research material relating to the experiences of families and care workers after the death of a person with dementia, as this is in keeping with the relatively recent interest in end of life care. The work that does exist mainly focuses on families' experiences of caring and demonstrates the range of emotions families face upon the death of the person with dementia and the grief process experienced.

Help and support is available from many third-sector organisations.

Organisations that can provide support

There is support for grief and bereavement. In the UK important support can be provided from:

Age UK Dementia Support Services

Bereavement, coping with the death of a loved one www.ageuk.org.uk/globalassets/age-uk/documents/information-guides/ageukig32_bereavement_inf.pdf

Coping with bereavement www.ageuk.org.uk/information-advice/health-wellbeing/relationships-family/bereavement/

End of life planning www.ageuk.org.uk/information-advice/money-legal/end-of-life-planning/.

Alzheimer's Society fact sheet on grief

www.alzheimers.org.uk/sites/default/files/pdf/factsheet_grief_
loss_and_bereavement.pdf

Carers National Association

www.carersuk.org/news-and-campaigns/features/hidden-
issues-when-caring-ends

Crossroads

Understanding End of Life Visions www.crossroadshospice.com/
hospice-palliative-care-blog/2017/july/19/understanding-
end-of-life-visions/

A Guide to Understanding End-of-Life Signs and Symptoms
www.crossroadshospice.com/hospice-caregiver-support/
end-of-life-signs/

Preparing for the Death of a Parent www.crossroadshospice.com/
hospice-caregiver-support/end-of-life-signs/death-of-a-
parent/

Grief Support Groups from Crossroads www.crossroadshospice.
com/grief-support/

The Journey After – A Bereavement Guide www.crossroadshospice.
com/grief-support/journey-after-booklet/

Cruse Bereavement

www.cruse.org.uk/

MacMillan

At the End of Life, Coping with Bereavement www.macmillan.
org.uk/information-and-support/coping/at-the-end-of-life/
coping-with-bereavement

Bereavement www.macmillan.org.uk/information-and-support/
oesophageal-gullet-cancer/coping/at-the-end-of-life/after-
death/bereavement.html#46795

NHS Bereavement Support

www.nhs.uk/conditions/stress-anxiety-depression/coping-with-
bereavement/

TIDE

Living Grief and Bereavement – A Booklet for Carers of People with Dementia www.tide.uk.net/wp-content/uploads/2019/11/05596-Grief-and-Bereavment-Booklet-for-carers.pdf

This chapter has explored the concepts of palliative and end of life care. Even when ACPs are in place, there are challenges that families and care professionals may face when providing end of life care, with particular reference to decision making and pain, nutrition and hydration issues. There are now policy directives and guidelines to advise on the delivery of end of life care to people living with dementia, but the research demonstrates that people do not always find themselves in situations where their wishes are upheld. There is an imperative to provide care that is sensitive and responsive to the needs of people with dementia who are dying – wherever they may be and whatever their degree of illness. This means we need to consider issues such as recognition and management of pain, and also the spiritual, emotional and cultural needs of both people with dementia who are dying and their families and friends.

REFERENCES

Allen, B. (ed.) (2002) *Religious Practice and People with Dementia: A Resource for Carers*. Newcastle: Christian Council on Ageing.

Alzheimer Society (2012) *My Life Until the End: Dying Well with Dementia*. www.alzheimers.org.uk/sites/default/files/migrate/downloads/my_life_until_the_end_dying_well_with_dementia.pdf

Badger, F., Clifford, C., Hewison, A. and Thomas, K. (2009) An evaluation of the implementation of a programme to improve end-of-life care in nursing homes. Palliative Medicine 23:502–511.

Brorson, H., Plymoth, H., Örmon, K. and Bolmsjö, I. (2014) Pain relief at the end of life: Nurses' experiences regarding end-of-life pain relief in patients with dementia. *Pain Management Nursing* 15(1), 315–323. doi.org/10.1016/j.pmn.2012.10.005

Brown, D. (2011) Pain assessment with cognitively impaired older people in the acute hospital setting. *British Journal of Pain* 5(3):18–22. doi: 10.1177/204946371100500305

Buiting, H., van Delden, J., Rietjens, J., Onwuteaka-Philipsen, B., Bilsen, J., Fischer, S., Lofmark, R., Miccinesi, G., Norup, M. and van der Heide, A. (2007) Forgoing artificial nutrition or hydration in patients nearing death in six European countries. *Journal of Pain and Symptom Management* 34(3):305–314.

Burns, C.M., Abernethy, A.P. and Dal Grande, E. (2013) Uncovering an invisible network of direct caregivers at the end of life: A population study. *Palliative Medicine* 27(7):608–615.

Connelly, A., Samspon, E.L. and Purandare, N. (2012) End-of-life care for people with dementia from ethnic minority groups: A systematic review. *Journal of the American Geriatric Society*. doi: 10.1111/j.1532-5415.2011.03754.x

Davies, N., Maio, L., Rait, G. and Iliffe, S. (2014) Quality end-of-life care for dementia: What have family carers told us so far? A narrative synthesis. *Palliative Medicine*. doi: 10.1177/0269216314526766

Davies, N., Manthorpe, J., Sampson, E.L., Lamahewa, K., Wilcock, J. and Matthew, R. (2018) Guiding practitioners through end of life care for people with dementia: The use of heuristics. *PloS One* 13(11). doi: 10.1371/journal.pone.0206422

Davies, N., Rait, G., Maio, L. and Iliffe, S. (2017) Family caregivers' conceptualisation of quality end-of-life care for people with dementia: A qualitative study. *Palliative Medicine* 31(8):726–733. doi: 10.1177/0269216316673552

Davis, C. (2007) Complex end-of-life care: Cultural issues. *European Journal of Palliative Care* 14(3):1–3–104.

Dekkers, W. (2004) Autonomy and the lived body in cases of severe dementia. In Purtillo, R. and ten Have, H. (Eds.), *Ethical Foundations of Palliative Care for Alzheimer's Disease*. Baltimore: The John Hopkins University Press (Chapter 7, pp. 115–130).

Dening, K.H., Jones, L. and Sampson, E.L. (2011) Advance care planning for people with dementia: A review. *International Psychogeriatrics* 23(10):1535–1551.

Department of Health (2008) *End of Life Care Strategy Promoting High Quality Care for All Adults at the End of Life*. London: Department of Health. https://webarchive.nationalarchives.gov.uk/20130104214035/www.dh.gov.uk/prod_consum_dh/groups/dh_digitalassets/@dh/@en/documents/digitalasset/dh_086345.pdf

De Roo, M.L., van der Steen, J.T., Galindo Garre, F., Van Den Noortgate, N., Onwuteaka-Philipsen, B.D., Deliens, L. and Francke, A.L. (2014) When do people with dementia die peacefully? An analysis of data collected prospectively in long-term care settings. *Palliative Medicine* 28(3):210–219. doi: 10.1177/0269216313509128

Froggatt, K., Vaughan, S., Bernard, C. and Wild, D. (2008) *Advance Care Planning in Care Homes for Older People: A Survey of Current Practice*. Lancaster: Lancaster University and IOELC.

Glass, A. (2016) Family caregiving and the site of care: Four narratives about end of life care for individuals with dementia. *Journal Social Work and End of Life Palliative Care* 12(1–2):23–46.

Goodman, C., Evans, C., Wilcock, J., et al. (2010) End of life care for community dwelling older people with dementia: An integrated review. *International Journal of Geriatric Psychiatry* 25(4):329–337.

Hill, S.R., Mason, H., Poole, M., Vale, L. and Robinson, L. (2017) What is important at the end of life for people with dementia? The views of people with dementia and their carers. *International Journal of Geriatric Psychiatry* 32(9):1037–1045. doi: 10.1002/gps.4564

Hirakawa, Y., Masuda, Y., Kuzuya, M., et al. (2006) End-of-life experience of demented elderly patients at home: Findings from DEATH project. *Psychogeriatrics* 6(2):60–67.

Ho, J.Q., Nguyen, C.D., Lopes, R., Ezeji-Okoye, S.C. and Kuschner, W.G. (2017) Spiritual care in the intensive care unit: A narrative review. *Journal of Intensive Care Medicine*. doi: 10.1177/0885066617712677

Horgas, A.L., Nichols A.L., Schapson, C.A. and Vietes, K. (2007) Assessing pain in persons with dementia: Relationships between the NOPPAIN, self-report, and behavioral observations. *Pain Management Nursing* 8:77–85.

Jolley, D., Benbow, S.M., Grizzell, M., Willmott, S., Bawn, S. and Kingston, P. (2010) Spirituality and faith in dementia. *Dementia*. doi.org/10.1177/1471301210370645

Jotkowitz, A.B., Clarfield, A.M. and Glick, S. (2005) The care of patients with dementia: A modern jewish ethical perspective. *Journal of the American Geriatrics Society* 53(5):881–884. doi.org/10.1111/j.1532-5415.2005.53271

Kumar, C.T.S. and Kuriakose, J.R. (2013) End-of-life care issues in advanced dementia. *Mental Health in Family Medicine* 10(3):129–132.

Kwok, T., Twinn, S. and Yan, E. (2007) The attitudes of Chinese family caregivers of older people with dementia towards life sustaining treatments. *Journal of Advanced Nursing* 58(3):256–262.

Lawrence, V., Samsi, K., Murray, J., Harari, D. and Banerjee, S. (2011) Dying well with dementia: Qualitative examination of end-of-life care. *British Journal Psychiatry* 199:417–422.

Lloyd-Williams, M., Dening, K.H. and Crowther, J. (2017) Dying with dementia-how can we improve the care and support of patients and their families. *Annals of Palliative Medicine* 6(4):306–309.

McAuliffe, L., Brown, B.D. and Fetherstonhaugh, D. (2012) Pain and dementia: An overview of the literature. *International Journal of Older People Nursing* 7:219–226. doi:10.1111/j.1748-3743.2012.00331.x

McParland, P., Kelly, F. and Innes, A. (2017) Dichotomising dementia: Is there another way? *Sociology of Health and Illness* 39(2):258–269.

Miranda, R., Bunn, F., Lynch, J., Van den Block, L. and Goodman, C. (2019) Palliative care for people with dementia living at home: A systematic review of interventions. *Palliative Medicine* 33(7):726–742. doi:10.1177/0269216319847092

Mogan, C., Lloyd-Williams, M., Dening, K.H. and Dowrick, C. (2018) The facilitators and challenges of dying at home with dementia: A narrative synthesis. *Palliative Medicine* 32(6):1042–1054. doi: 10.1177/0269216318760442

Moon, F., McDermott, F. and Kissane, D. (2018) Systematic review for the quality of end-of-life care for patients with dementia in the hospital setting. *American Journal of Hospice and Palliative Medicine*. doi: 10.1177/1049909118776985

National Council for Palliative Care Dementia (2014) *Dementia Roadmap.* https://dementiaroadmap.info/category/dying-well/#.XeZWkzD7R1s

National Dementia Intelligence Network and National End of Life Care Intelligence Network (2016) *Dying with Dementia Briefing.* London: Public Health England. https://assets.publishing.service.gov.uk/government/uploads/system/uploads/attachment_data/file/733064/Dying_with_dementia_briefing.pdf

North West Coast Strategic Clinical Network (2018) *Palliative Care Guidelines In Dementia* (2nd edition). NHS England. www.england.nhs.uk/north/wp-content/uploads/sites/5/2018/06/palliative-care-guidelines-in-dementia.pdf

Nuffield Council on Bioethics (2009) *Dementia: Ethical Issues, a Guide to the Report.* www.nuffieldbioethics.org/fileLibrary/pdf/Nuffield_Dementia_short_guide_FINAL.pdf

Pinch, W. (2004) Advance directives and end-of-life decision making in Alzheimer disease. In Purtillo, R. and ten Have, H. (Eds.), *Ethical Foundations of Palliative Care for Alzheimer Disease.* Baltimore: John Hopkins University Press.

Sampson, E.L., Burns, A. and Richards, M. (2011) Improving end-of-life care for people with dementia. *British Journal of Psychiatry* 199(5):357–359.

Sampson, E.L., Candy, B. and Jones, L. (2009) Enteral tube feeding for older people with advanced dementia. *Cochrane Database Systematic Review.* 15(2):CD007209. doi: 10.1002/14651858. CD007209.pub2

Sellars, M., Chung, O., Nolte, L., Tong, A., Pond, D., Fetherstonhaugh, D., Mcinerney, F., Sinclair, C. and Detering, K.M. (2019) Perspectives of people with dementia and carers on advance care planning and end-of-life care: A systematic review and thematic synthesis of qualitative studies. *Palliative Medicine.* doi: 10.1177/0269216318809571

Slape, J. (2014) Dementia and palliative care: The spiritual needs of family members. *Journal of Religion, Spirituality and Ageing*:215–230. doi: 10.1080/15528030.2013.830237

Small, N., Froggatt, K. and Downs, M. (2007) *Living and Dying with Dementia: Dialogues about Palliative Care.* Oxford: Oxford University Press.

Social Care Institute for Excellence (SCIE) (2015) *End of Life Care in Dementia: An Introduction.* www.scie.org.uk/dementia/advanced-dementia-and-end-of-life-care/end-of-life-care/introduction. asp?gclid=CjwKCAiArJjvBRACEiwA-Wiqq3_fs9ZTyR20OWIdieC-Vn_SiV37_QYGGW8qJv8joJRcTSn1JHuDchoCGPcQAvD_BwE

Thune-Boyle, I., Sampson, E., Jones, L., King, M., Lee, D. and Blanchard, M. (2010) Challenges to improving end of life care of people with advanced dementia in the UK. Dementia 9(2):259–284.

TIDE and DEEP (2018) *End of Life Care and Post Bereavement Support: Shifting the Conversation from Difficult to Important Sharing the Perspectives of People Living with Dementia and Their Carers.* http://www.innovationsindementia.org.uk/wp-content/uploads/2018/09/End-of-Life-Care-Post-Bereavement-Support-Shifting-the-Conversation-from-Difficult-to-Important41.pdf

Torjesen, I. (2013) Bad press over Liverpool care pathway has scared patients and doctors, say experts. *British Medical Journal* 346:f175. doi: 10.1136/bmj.f175 23305844

Wernham, C., Jordan, A. and Hughes, J.C. (2018) Assessing pain in dementia: Tools or tacit knowledge (or both)? *British Journal of General Practice* 68(669):196–197. https://doi.org/10.3399/bjgp18X695657

CONCLUSION

Dementia is a complex condition that impacts on individuals with the diagnosis differently at different points in time. In this book we have charted the journey of dementia, from pre-diagnosis to diagnosis, to post-diagnostic support, to care transitions that occur alongside increasing care and support needs, to end of life, this is summarized in Figure 0.1. The dementia journey will be experienced differently by different people, influenced by changes in practices and policy directives over time, but also due to the individuality of each person living with dementia and those who provide them with care and support. The context leading up to the diagnosis (discussed in chapters 1 and 2) can lay the foundations for later experiences. Delays in receiving the diagnosis impact on the adjustment process and the possibilities to develop advance directives or care plans (discussed in chapter 7) and the opportunity to

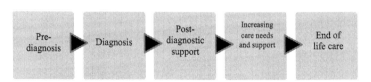

Figure 0.1 The Dementia Journey

meet others with the diagnosis who may be going through similar issues and who can share their strategies for adjusting to the challenges dementia can bring to everyday life.

The personal accounts throughout this book from Gail (in chapters 1, 2, 4, 5, 6 and 7), written about her experiences of caring for her mother and then her father, demonstrate how things can develop over time in terms of support available and the approach of professionals. Lesley's personal accounts throughout this book (chapters 1, 2, 3, 5, 6 and 7) help us understand the experience of living with dementia, one in which she must recognise that her stated preferences may not be possible to meet as changes occur for both herself and her family.

Dementia is not an easy experience for anyone. There are, however, things that can be done to help navigate the journey and to support both the person living with dementia and their family members along the way, as our examples of providing post-diagnostic support in section 2 of this book illustrate. Some of these are common sense and may at first sight appear easy and obvious, but the experiences of Gail and Lesley, and many other people living with dementia who have shared their experiences in the research literature, show that the solutions that could help are not always available. This can be simply the attitude of a taxi driver as Lesley highlights via her experiences (chapter 3) or the availability of services as Gail's account illustrates (chapter 4), that would enable family members to provide support and care in the ways that they would prefer.

Policies, strategies and plans to support the development and delivery of high-quality care for people living with dementia and their families exist worldwide (Alzheimer Disease International, 2019). Guidelines have also been developed to help countries develop and implement such plans (WHO, 2018). Existing plans and guides provide recognition that all plans need to lead to impact and clearly provide a platform to move what can be the rhetoric of policy to actions that will benefit people living with dementia globally. However, if we look at particular examples, such as end of life (chapter 7) where many policies and guides now exist, the reality for people living with dementia and their families may still not reflect the ideals and principles that have been carefully and thoughtfully developed. This may in part be due to the stressful and emotional aspects of end of life care, but it may also be due to staff and service shortages. Despite knowledge that people living with dementia and their families would prefer for the person with dementia to remain at home until their death, this is actually rarely the case – the majority of people living with dementia do not die at home.

Great strides have been made in the dementia field over the last two decades. The move to ensure that the voices of people living with dementia are heard has helped to shape the agendas of policy and practice. However, there is more to be done. Raising awareness of dementia amongst the general public has been identified as key and lobbying groups such as the Alzheimer's Societies of individual countries, Alzheimer Europe and Alzheimer Disease International have all helped to raise awareness of dementia, reduce stigma and support earlier diagnosis. This is important as it is at this early point in the symptoms of dementia when some of the anti-dementia medications may help and when the person and their family can plan for the future together. Encouraging opportunities for earlier approaches for help and advice, perhaps through screening and proactive identification via routine health appointments, may help identify dementia earlier and enable supports to be put in place as early as possible to promote living well with dementia.

The experience of diagnosis is one that is fraught for all concerned. Although a diagnostic label may bring relief (there is actually something wrong, it's not just our imagination), it also then begins a journey of learning about what support is available, adapting to the changing abilities of the person with dementia, taking on different roles to provide suitable support and, as Gail and Lesley's personal accounts demonstrate (chapters 3, 4 and 5), sometimes a battle to get the help and support they would like. There are many examples of innovative practice in dementia, but these vary from country to country and within countries. Some of this is understandable, and the individual cultural context is important to recognise; however, there are also common support needs that people living with dementia and their families have at different points along the dementia journey.

The challenge, as we see it, is to move beyond the policy and guidelines until we reach a point where the lived experiences of the person diagnosed and those that support them is optimal. Alzheimer Disease International (2019, 6) sets out the following priority action areas for all countries to achieve:

- Dementia as a public health priority.
- Dementia awareness and friendliness.

- Dementia risk reduction.
- Dementia diagnosis, treatment, care and support.
- Support for dementia carers.
- Information systems for dementia.
- Dementia research and innovation.

We are perhaps further ahead now than ever before in having an international consensus about what needs to be achieved in the dementia field to bring about impactful change that will make a positive difference to the lives of those with dementia and their families.

We recognise, as do the people living with dementia and family members that we have worked with over the years, that each individual has unique needs that may not always be able to be fully met. However, they also want to be treated with dignity at all times, from pre-diagnosis to end of life; given time by professionals and society generally, for example to accommodate the changes to the speed that they may be able to process information; given access to appropriate support at the right time for them; and to be given access to opportunities to enhance their lives and sense of wellbeing throughout their journey with dementia.

People living with dementia and their families are often frustrated when services and supports they have accessed that they feel benefit them end, due to time-limited and short-term funding. Lesley's experience of the dementia-friendly swimming sessions exemplify this. She learnt how to swim when she had dementia, and built up her skill in this area of her life that led her to feel well and physically strong, but then this initiative ended. We are sure that you will also have come across examples of excellent local initiatives ending due to changes in funding priorities, or projects that were time limited. Despite evidence that they 'work' for participants, they still come to an end. Although any support that makes a difference, even if for a short time, is positive, there is a question about the ethics of removing services from people who rely on them to live well and to live independently, or in the case of carers, that enable them to continue to provide support and care to their relatives or friends.

Adjusting to increased care and support needs is difficult for the individual with dementia and for families. Good ongoing monitoring and reviews of the needs of people living with dementia may help to avoid some 'crisis' points that can lead to care home placements or hospital stays. However it is important to recognise that these 'crisis' points will arise for some, perhaps if the primary carer becomes ill or the person with dementia develops another condition. This means that although the ideal of many may be to stay at home, this will not always be possible. As supports have improved to help maintain people living independently at home, those who do need care home or hospital placements may have complex care needs due to progressive dementia or from co-morbidities (different conditions/disease). Care in hospitals and care homes has been subject to much scrutiny and it is recognised that the work staff do is highly skilled and requires support for staff members via staff development and training opportunities to enable them to provide the high-quality support policy has directed people living with dementia and their families should expect to receive.

Our experiences as authors of the book, namely, as an academic researcher (Anthea), a person living with dementia (Lesley) and a family member (Gail), have shown that while support has improved for many people who are affected by dementia, there are still examples where people experience acute stress and care needs that are not met. Until we can be confident that all people living with dementia are fully supported to live as well as possible with dementia, then our efforts as individuals will continue to bring about change and improvements. We hope that in whatever capacity you are reading this book, be that as a person living with dementia, a family member, a student on a course, a health and social care professional, a researcher or in some other role, that you join us in working to achieve an outcome where the basics of dementia care throughout the dementia journey become a reality for all.

REFERENCES

Alzheimer Disease International (2019) *From Plan to Impact II: The Urgent Need for Action*. London: ADI. www.alz.co.uk/adi/pdf/from-plan-to-impact-2019.pdf

WHO (2018) *Towards a Dementia Plan: A WHO Guide*. World Health Organisation. https://apps.who.int/iris/bitstream/handle/10665/272642/9789241514132-eng.pdf?ua=1

INDEX

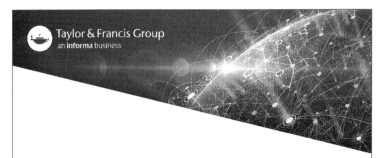